Genes and Cancer

Edited by Guy-Joseph Lemamy

Published in London, United Kingdom

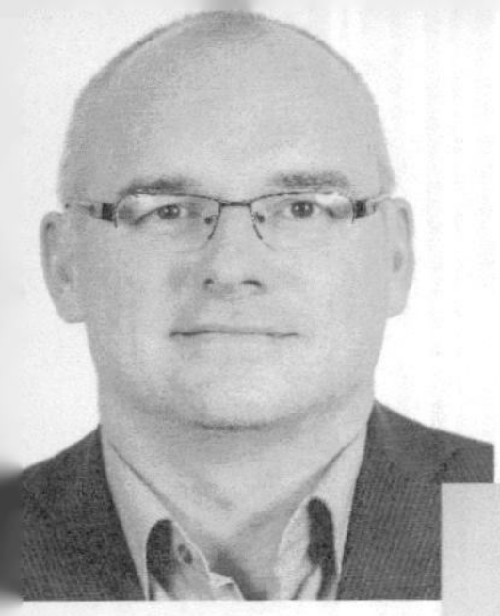
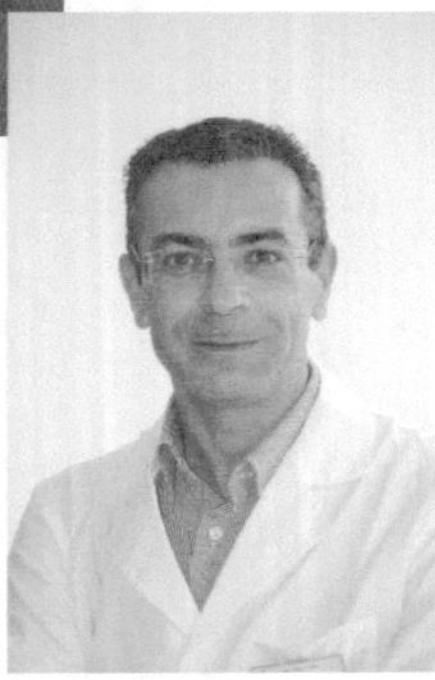
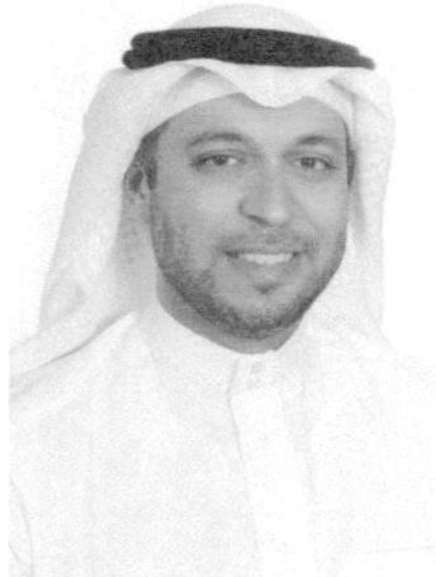
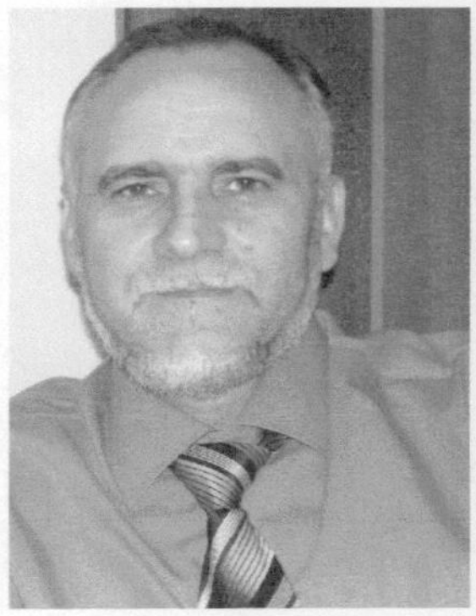
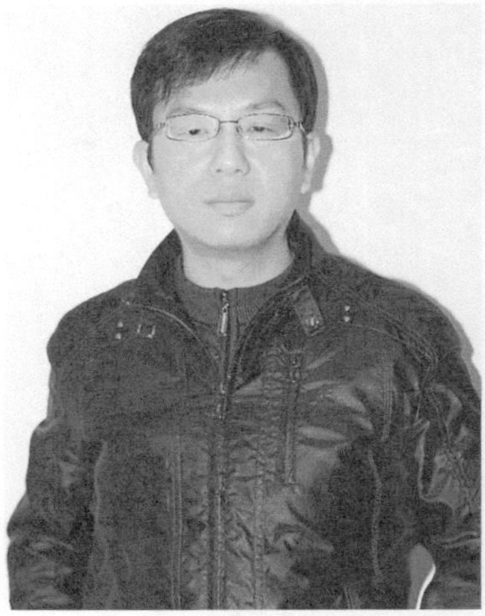
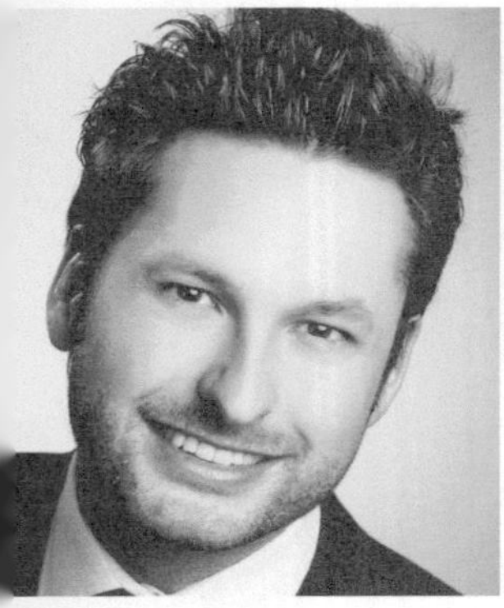
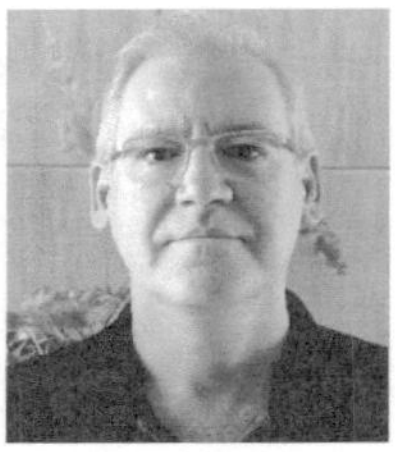

IntechOpen

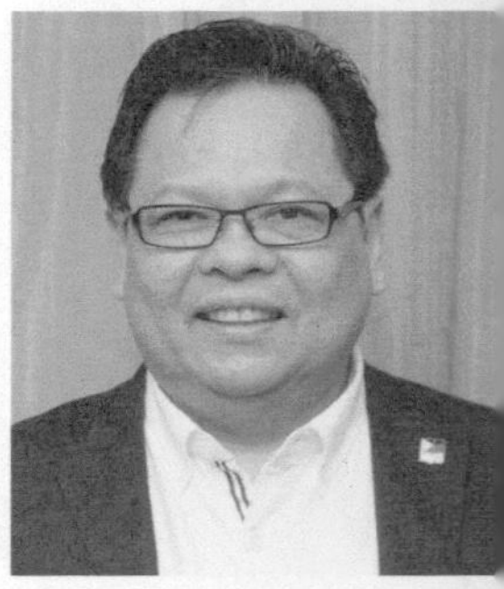
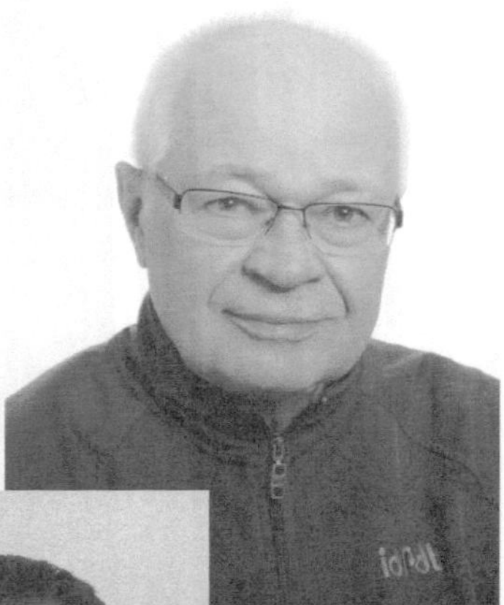
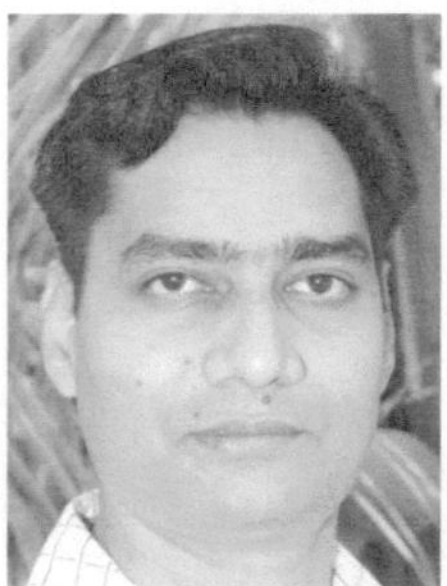
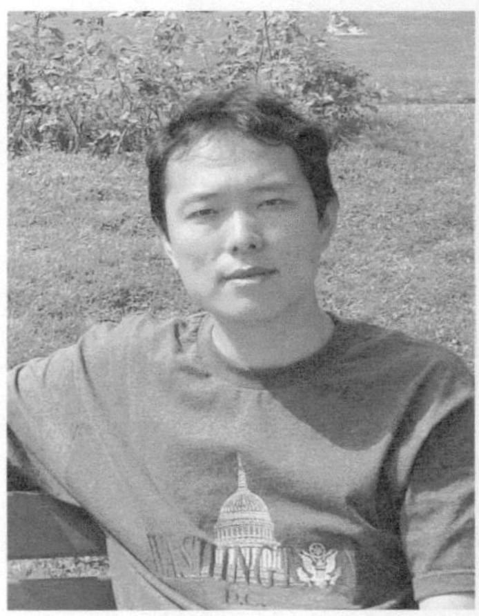
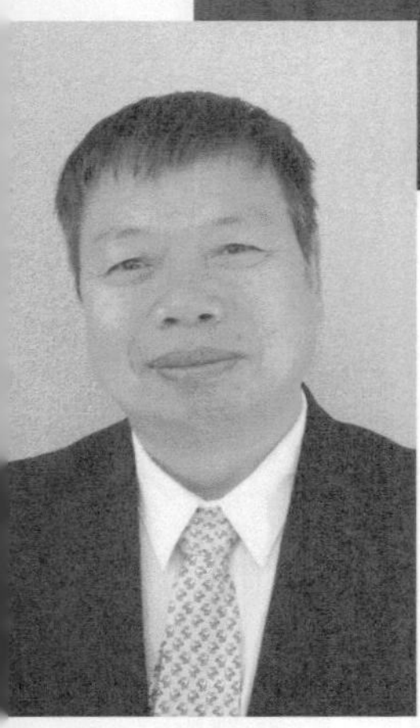
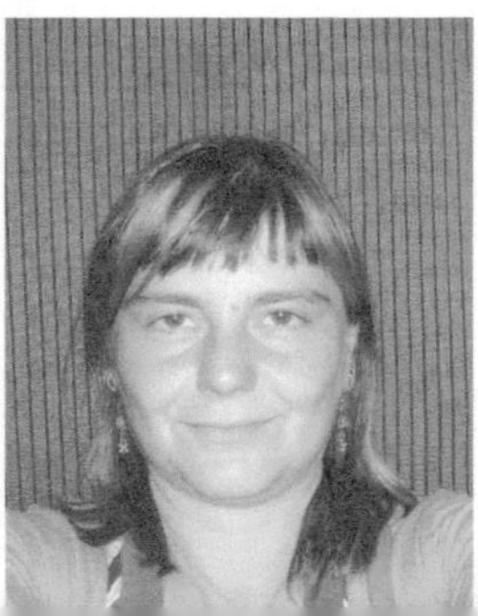

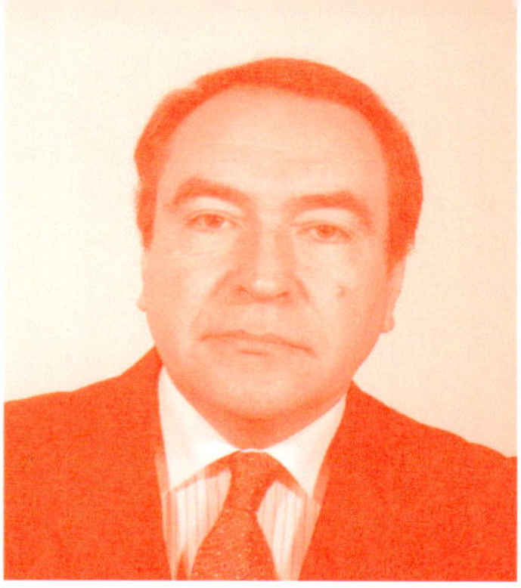
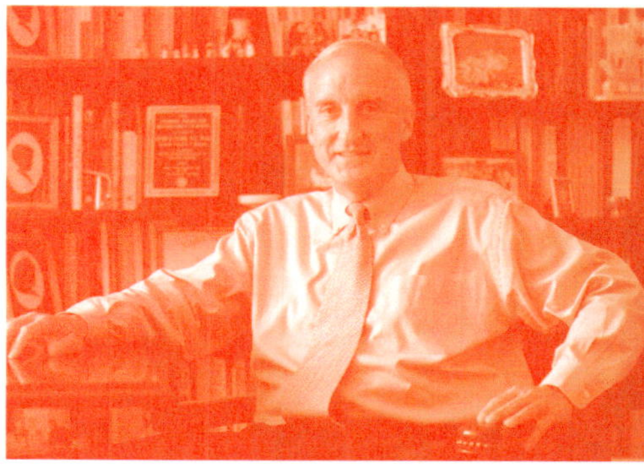
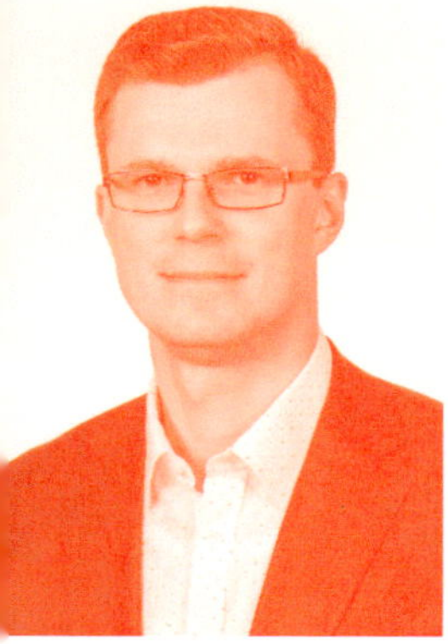
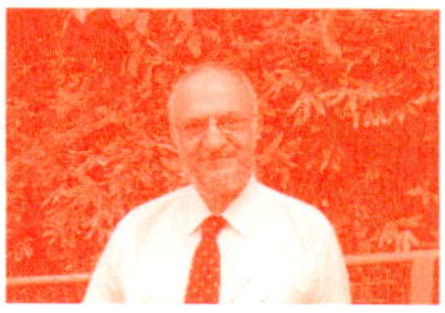
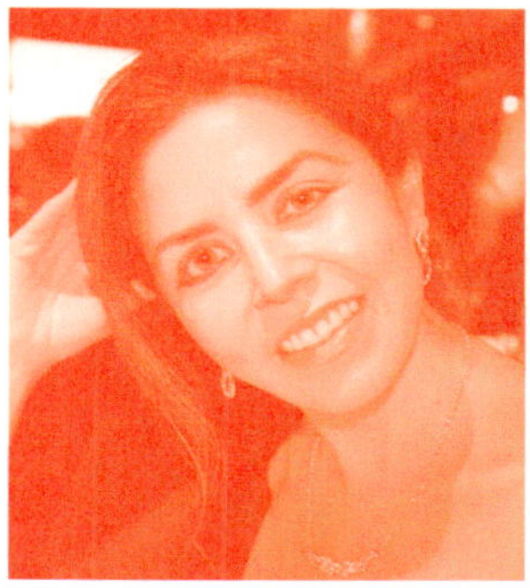

Supporting open minds since 2005

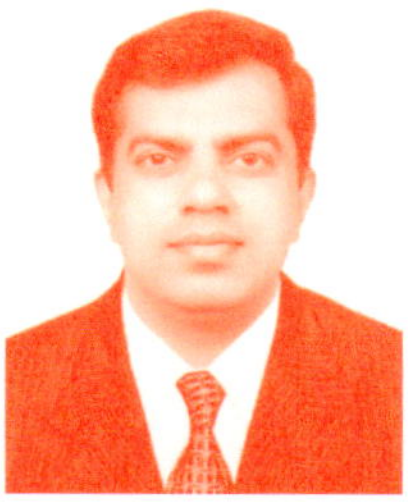
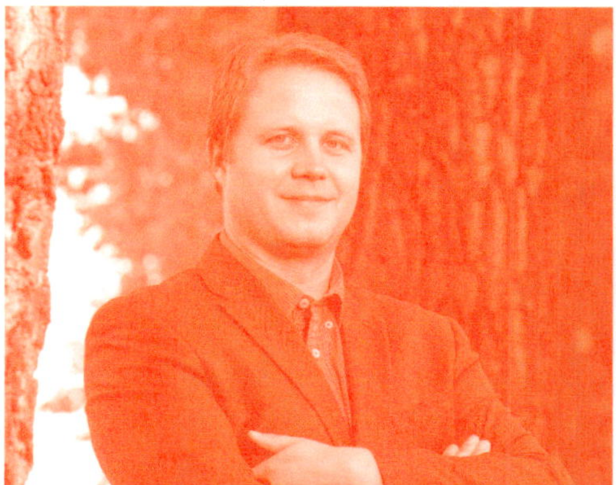
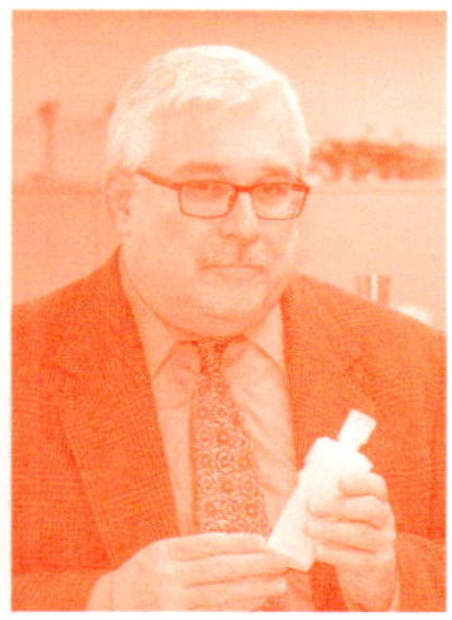
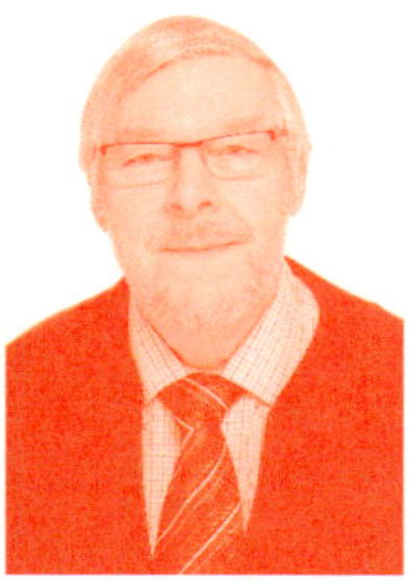
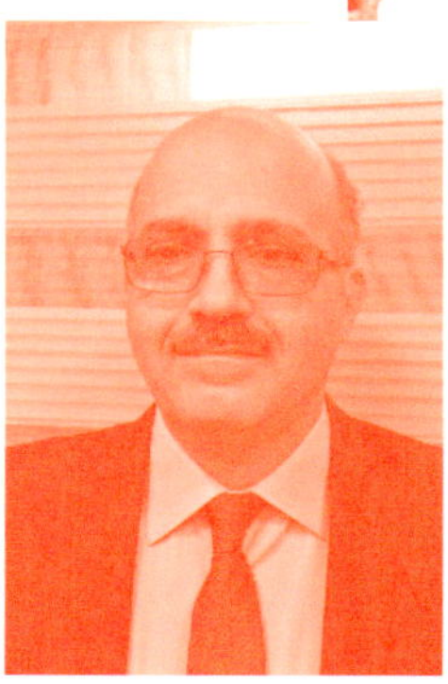
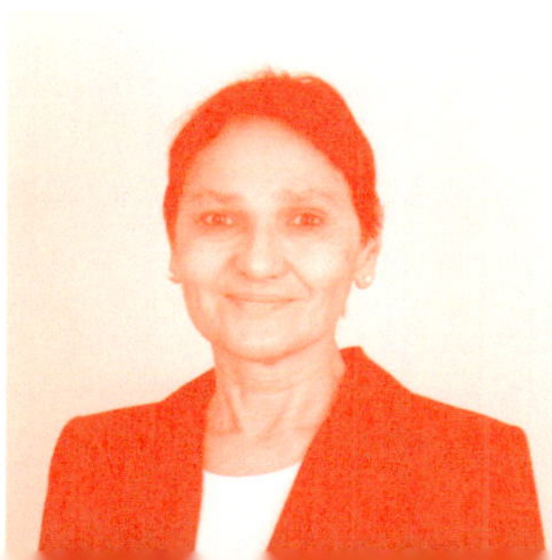
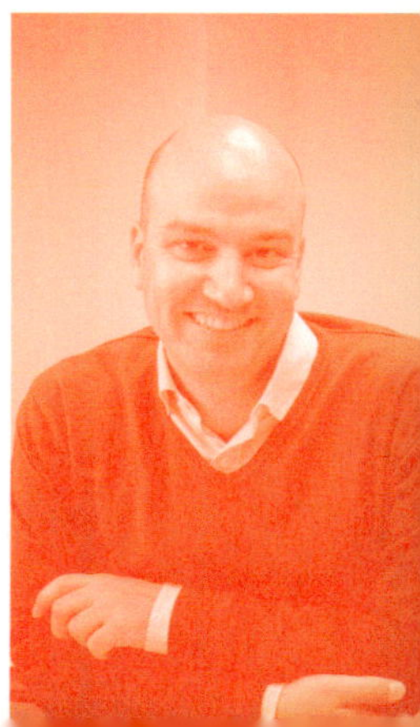

Genes and Cancer
http://dx.doi.org/10.5772/intechopen.78120
Edited by Guy-Joseph Lemamy

Contributors
Wan Lam, Mateus Camargo Barros-Filho, Florian Guisier, Leigha Rock, Daiana Becker-Santos, Adam Sage, Erin Marshall, Guang-Jer Wu, Leopold F. Fröhlich, Maria Mrakovcic, Jian Zhang, Xia Li, Liangliang Shen, Yan Li, Libo Yao, Amal Qattan

First published in London, United Kingdom, 2019 by IntechOpen
IntechOpen is the global imprint of INTECHOPEN LIMITED, registered in England and Wales, registration number: 11086078, The Shard, 25th floor, 32 London Bridge Street
London, SE19SG - United Kingdom
Printed in Croatia

British Library Cataloguing-in-Publication Data
A catalogue record for this book is available from the British Library

Additional hard and PDF copies can be obtained from orders@intechopen.com

Genes and Cancer
Edited by Guy-Joseph Lemamy
p. cm.
Print ISBN 978-1-78984-426-9
Online ISBN 978-1-78984-427-6
eBook (PDF) ISBN 978-1-83881-974-3

For EU product safety concerns:
IN TECH d.o.o., Prolaz Marije Krucifikse Kozulić 3, 51000 Rijeka, Croatia, info@intechopen.com or visit our website at intechopen.com.

Meet the editor

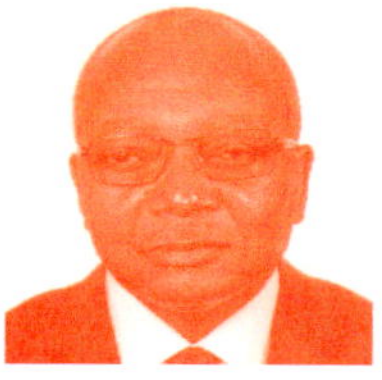

Guy Joseph Lemamy, PhD, is currently a professor in the Department of Cellular and Molecular Biology-Genetics, and Director of the Laboratory of Cellular and Molecular Biopathologies, at the Faculty of Medicine, Université des Sciences de la Santé, Libreville, Gabon. He was a member of the Scientific Advisory Board of Gabon Scientific Research Guiding Plan. Dr. Lemamy obtained his PhD in Biochemistry and Cell Biology at the Faculty of Medicine, Université Montpellier 1, France. His PhD thesis concerned tumor markers in breast cancer, led by the Medical Research Institute (INSERM U148) in Montpellier, France. Dr. Lemamy is editor of world-class books in the field of cancer research and author of many book chapters and journal articles on tumor markers.

Contents

Preface

Cancer is a malignant tumor caused by DNA damage, which leads to uncontrolled cell growth. Tumor progression is locally favored by the mitogenic effects of hormones or growth factors, which stimulate the tumor's growth, or the activation of vascular endothelial growth factor receptor, which induces angiogenesis and leads to metastasis. About 300 out of 25,000 genes that set up the human genome are involved in cancer pathology. These genes are divided into three groups: oncogenes, tumor suppressor genes, and DNA repair genes. Activated oncogenes promote the development of cancer, whereas the tumor suppressor and DNA repair genes have a protective role by respectively inhibiting cell cycle progression and inducing apoptosis, or by repairing DNA damage occurring during the cell cycle.

The purpose of this book is to discuss the topics of tumor suppressor genes and add to knowledge of the understanding of cancer using advanced biochemistry, cell, and molecular biology tools. Tumor suppressor genes can be used as targets of preventive therapy, markers of risk that can be used to identify populations at high risk, or markers of a drug's toxicity used in prevention, which can help to monitor its tolerance.

The book is divided in three sections and five chapters.

Section I: Studies of Potential Tumor Suppressor Genes (Chapter 1: N-Myc Downstream-Regulated Gene 2 (NDRG2) as a Novel Tumor Suppressor in Multiple Human Cancers; Chapter 2: METCAM/MUC18: A Novel Tumor Suppressor for Some Cancers).

Section II: Genes with Dual Suppressor and Oncogenic Activities (Chapter 3: Tumor Suppressor Genes with Oncogenic Roles in Lung Cancer; Chapter 4: Duplicitous Disposition of Micro-RNAs (miRs) in Breast Cancer).

Section III: Tumor Suppressor Proteins in Cell Signaling Pathways (Chapter 5: Regulation of HDACi-triggered Autophagy by the Tumor Suppressor Protein p53).

The first chapter discusses the role of the N-myc Downregulated Gene 2 (NDRG2) as a tumor suppressor gene in multiple cancers. *In vitro* and *in vivo* studies report cancer cell inhibition, metastasis cell differentiation, and cell cycle arrest mediated by NDRG2. The authors suggest that NDRG2 might be considered as a potential target for cancer therapeutics and treatment. However, the detailed mechanism requires further investigation to confirm its tumor suppressor function.

The role of METCAM/MUC18 as a possible tumor suppressor gene is reported in Chapter 2. METCAM/MUC18 is a cell adhesion molecule (CAM) that belongs to the Ig-like gene superfamily and is located in the human 11q23-3 chromosome. Multiple studies have shown evidence that METCAM/MUC18 might play a tumor suppressor role in many cancers, including mouse melanoma and human nasopharyngeal, ovarian, prostate, colorectal, hemangioma, and pancreatic cancers. Moreover, in some cancers such as nasopharyngeal cancers, METCAM/MUC18 plays a dual suppressor and promoter role. Thereby, the authors suggest that METCAM/MUC18 could be used as a new therapeutics target for such cancer treatment.

In the third chapter the authors discuss the issue of tumor suppressor genes with dual suppressive and oncogenic roles in lung cancer. Among such genes, TP53 (a well-known tumor suppressor gene in many cancers) activating alterations can promote cancer development and progression, despite its classic functions of cell cycle regulation, DNA repair, senescence, and apoptosis, which give it the role of "guardian of the genome." The authors also describe the role of nuclear factor 1B (NF1B), which belongs to a transcription factor family, including NF1A, NF1B, NF1C, and NF1X. These transcription factors lead to DNA repression or activation of genes in a context-specific manner. NF1B in particular has been described as both an oncogene and a potential tumor suppressor gene. It is amplified and/or overexpressed in many types of cancers such as melanoma, breast and esophagus cancers, and in salivary glands. A lower expression of NF1B is associated with shorter average survival, less-differentiated tumor features, and repressed expression of cell differentiation markers in lung adenocarcinoma. A tumor suppressive role of NF1B has been suggested in non-small cell lung cancer. NOTCH is another gene acting as an oncogene in lung adenocarcinoma and has a potential role as a tumor suppressor gene. The authors also report the tumor suppressive functions of NKX2-1 in lung adenocarcinoma. This gene acts in the restriction of cell motility, invasion, and metastatic ability. The dual role of NKX2-1 depends on EGFR, KRAS, and TP53 status in lung adenocarcinoma. NKX2-1 acts by enhancing EGFR-driven tumorigenesis. Another gene with a dual role is the Metastasis-Associated Lung Adenocarcinoma Transcript 1 (MALAT1). This gene has been previously identified as an oncogenic transcript and considered as a marker of metastasis, poor patient survival, and chemotherapy resistance in non-small cell lung cancer. MALAT1 promotes carcinogenesis through p53 deacetylation and enhances cell migration. In contrast, MALAT1 has been shown to reduce invasiveness in PTEN-expressing tumors. For example, MALAT1 reduces invasiveness of cerebral metastasis by sustaining the blood–brain barrier.

In the fourth chapter, the author provides an overview of the role of microRNAs (miRNAs) in breast cancer. The miRNAs are highly conserved in humans but are not translated into proteins. However, these molecules are involved in gene regulation and carcinogenesis. The miRNAs have dual roles in cancer pathology. Several miRNAs are both cancer and tissue specific. Because the primary role of miRNAs is to decrease target mRNA expression, they are upregulated by cancer cells aren, often those that support cancer growth and are called oncomirs. Other miRNAs are downregulated and referred to as tumor suppressor miRNAs. Since miRNAs are released by cancer cells in the blood, the author concludes by suggesting that both monitoring and targeting miRNAs enables the diagnosis and monitoring of breast cancer as well as the opportunity for the development of novel therapeutics.

Studies in the fifth and final chapters report regulation by the tumor suppressor protein p53, the most common tumor suppressor gene, of autophagy mediated by histone deacetylase inhibitors (HDACi) in cancer cells. The authors refer to the cellular mechanism of autophagy and describe biological signaling pathways regulated by tumor suppressor protein p53 in the formation of autophagosomes, the HDACi-induced cell death.

I am grateful to the IntechOpen Access Publisher team for giving me the opportunity to be the editor of this book. I am particularly thankful to Ms. Ivana Barac, the Publishing Process Manager, for guiding me through the publication process and coordinating the different steps. I would like to thank all the authors who have contributed to this book by writing their chapters and for making my requested revisions to them. I also thank them for sharing their knowledge of the understanding of carcinogenesis surrounding the issue of tumor suppressor genes. I dedicate this book to all my colleagues and students at Université des Sciences de la Santé of Libreville, Gabon. Lastly, I would like to thank my family for their support throughout my academic career, particularly Jeanne-Otoua, Marie-Thérèse Moungala, and my wife Sophie-Mindili for their understanding during this book project process.

Guy Joseph Lemamy, PhD
Professor and Head of Department of Cellular and
Molecular Biology-Genetics

Faculty of Medicine, University of Health Sciences
(Faculté de Médecine, Université des Sciences de la Santé),
Libreville, Gabon

Section 1

Studies of Potential Tumor Suppressor Genes

Chapter 1

N-Myc Downstream-Regulated Gene 2 (NDRG2) as a Novel Tumor Suppressor in Multiple Human Cancers

Jian Zhang, Xia Li, Liangliang Shen, Yan Li and Libo Yao

Abstract

N-myc downstream-regulated gene 2 (NDRG2) was identified as a novel tumor suppressor gene in regulating the proliferation, differentiation, apoptosis and metastasis of multiple cancer types. Consistent with this finding, we and other groups observed the decreased NDRG2 expression in multiple human cancer cell lines and tumors, including breast cancer, colorectal cancer, and cervical cancer. We identified NDRG2 as a stress sensor for hypoxia, DNA damage stimuli and endoplasmic reticulum stress (ERS). Our recent data showed that NDRG2 could promote the differentiation of colorectal cancer cells. Interestingly, we found that reduced NDRG2 expression was a powerful and independent predictor of poor prognosis of colorectal cancer patients. Furthermore, NDRG2 can inhibit epithelial-mesenchymal transition (EMT) by positively regulating E-cadherin expression. Moreover, NDRG2-deficient mice show spontaneous development of various tumor types, including T-cell lymphomas, providing in vivo evidence that NDRG2 functions as a tumor suppressor gene. We believe that NDRG2 is a novel tumor suppressor and might be a therapeutic target for cancer treatment.

Keywords: NDRG2, tumor suppressor, stress sensor, p53, differentiation, EMT, metastasis, cancer metabolism

1. The finding of NDRG2

The human NDRG2 sequence was first described by Deng et al. as a protein containing an acyl-carrier protein (ACP)-like domain [1, 2]. The gene was cloned from differentially expressed genes between glioblastoma and normal brain tissues using PCR-based subtractive hybridization in 2003 [2]. NDRG2, NDRG1, NDRG3, and NDRG4 comprise the NDRG gene family and share approximately 59–68% homology. Additionally, NDRG family members display over 92% homology between humans and mice [1].

We identified NDRG2 as a novel tumor suppressor gene that plays a role in regulating the proliferation, differentiation, apoptosis and metastasis of multiple types of malignant tumors [1, 2]. Consistent with this finding, NDRG2 downregulation has been observed in multiple human cancer cell lines and tumors [3–5]. Additionally, other groups later confirmed our finding [6, 7]. NDRG2 was identified as a stress sensor for hypoxia, DNA damage stimuli and endoplasmic reticulum stress (ERS), and could inhibit the proliferation and promote the differentiation of colorectal carcinoma cells [8]. Moreover, NDRG2-deficient mice show spontaneous development of various tumor types, providing in vivo evidence that NDRG2 functions as a tumor suppressor gene. In this chapter, we will introduce the recent findings of NDRG2 as tumor suppressor in vitro and in vivo, and also the detailed mechanism.

2. NDRG2 as a hypoxia and DNA damage responder

Our group firstly identified NDRG2 as a protein containing an acyl-carrier protein (ACP)-like domain. The gene was cloned from differentially expressed genes between glioblastoma and normal brain tissues using PCR-based subtractive hybridization in 2003. NDRG2, NDRG1, NDRG3, and NDRG4 comprise the NDRG gene family [1] and share approximately 59–68% homology. Additionally, NDRG family members display over 92% homology between humans and mice.

The expression and cellular localization of NDRG2 were altered following exposure to different stresses, supporting the role of NDRG2 as a cellular stress sensor. Wang et al. found that NDRG2 expression was markedly upregulated in several cancer cell lines exposed to hypoxic conditions or similar stresses at both the mRNA and protein levels [9]. Hypoxia-inducible factor-1α (HIF-1α) can directly bind to hypoxia response elements (HREs) in the NDRG2 promoter, thus upregulating NDRG2 expression under hypoxia. Importantly, enforcing the expression of NDRG2 can strongly increase the apoptosis of cancer cells. Alternatively, NDRG2 can translocate from the cytoplasm to the nucleus under DNA damage stress. However, no explicit nuclear localization signal (NLS) sequence has been identified in the NDRG2 protein. Although NLSs are the most common type of nuclear import elements, other mechanisms may also be involved in NDRG2 translocation. For example, Liu et al. and Cao et al. confirmed that NDRG2 was upregulated by p53 or adriamycin (ADR) treatment [10, 11]. Thus, NDRG2 can translocate into the nucleus and increase p53-dependent cell apoptosis through the DNA damage repair mechanism. Furthermore, we found that NDRG2 expression was decreased in ADR-resistant breast cancer cells. However, NDRG2 rescue could promote ADR sensitivity through inhibiting proliferation and promoting cellular damage responses and apoptosis in a p53-dependent manner. Interestingly, we found that NDRG2 upregulated Bad expression by increasing its half-life, which is associated with p53 expression in mitochondria. Thus, NDRG2 promoted the therapeutic sensitivity of breast cancer cells in a p53-dependent manner by preventing p53 from entering the nucleus to participate in DNA damage repair rather than by changing its expression [12].

We first found that NDRG2 is positively regulated by p53. The first intron of the NDRG2 gene contains a site that binds p53 directly and mediates wild-type (WT) p53-dependent transactivation [11]. In addition, NDRG2 enhances p53-mediated apoptosis, whereas overexpression of NDRG2 suppresses tumor cell growth independently of p53 mutation. NDRG2 enhances p53-mediated apoptosis of hepatocarcinoma cells by downregulating ERCC6 (also named cockayne syndrome B—CSB) expression, which is critical for nucleotide excision repair capacity [10]. Thus, excision repair cross-complementing complementation group 6 (ERCC6) is an NDRG2-inducible target gene that is involved in the p53-mediated apoptosis pathway.

3. NDRG2 functions as a novel ER stress-responsive protein and unfolded protein response (UPR) modulator

The ER is an essential organelle involved in many cellular processes, including protein folding and maturation, lipid synthesis and calcium homeostasis. When cells are challenged by different environmental or intracellular insults, such as energy or nutrient deficiency, hypoxia, or oxidative stresses, ER's function is disrupted, causing accumulation of unfolded or misfolded proteins in the ER, a condition which is defined as ER stress [13, 14]. This triggers integrated signaling pathways to deal with the unfolded proteins, a phenomenon known as the UPR, which operates to restore ER homeostasis or, alternatively, lead to cell death under prolonged or severe ER stress [13, 14].

The UPR contains three branches initiated by three ER-resident transmembrane sensors: protein kinase RNA-like ER kinase (PERK), inositol-requiring enzyme 1α (IRE1α), and activating transcription factor 6 (ATF6) [15]. ER stress and the UPR are intensively involved in not only physiological conditions but also the pathogenesis of many diseases, including cancer [14, 16]. Accumulating implicates ER stress and the UPR in different aspects of tumorigenesis and tumor progression.

NDRG2 is a stress-responsive gene [1], and our laboratory recently reported that as such, NDRG2 is implicated in ER stress [17] in addition to the hypoxia and DNA damage response. Different ER stress inducers, including thapsigargin (Tg), tunicamycin (Tm) and dithiothreitol (DTT), can induce NDRG2 mRNA and protein expression in human hepatoma SK-Hep-1 and HepG2 cells. In NDRG2-overexpressing hepatoma cell lines and Ndrg2 knockout (KO) mouse liver tissues, among the three UPR branches, NDRG2 interacts with PERK upon ER stress and facilitates PERK pathway activity, enhancing downstream ATF4 and CHOP activity. Thus, overexpression of NDRG2 promotes ERS-induced apoptosis, while silencing or knockdown of NDRG2 does the opposite, both in cell lines and in vivo. These data suggest that NDRG2 is a novel ER stress-responsive protein and an important component of the UPRosome, acting as a PERK cofactor to facilitate PERK branch signaling and thereby contributing to ER stress-induced apoptosis [17]. Therefore, apart from its already established role, NDRG2 could be considered a component of the UPRosome and a key player in cell fate decisions during ER stress. However, whether NDRG2 regulates PERK by affecting its dimer/oligomer status or its post-translational modification or by competing with other regulators for binding is worthy of further investigation.

4. NDRG2 as a novel prognostic biomarker in cancer

NDRG2 expression is mainly detected in the muscle, brain, heart, liver, colon [18]. Interestingly, NDRG2 expression is nearly undetectable in the thymus, the bone marrow, the testis, and peripheral blood leukocytes, suggesting an inverse correlation between the NDRG2 gene expression level and cell proliferation status [18–20]. We and other groups confirmed the pattern of decreased NDRG2 expression in tumors compared with normal tissues in cancers including glioma [2, 19, 21], colorectal cancer [8, 22, 23], breast cancer [3, 24], lung cancer [25], thyroid cancer [26, 27], myeloid leukemia [28, 29] oral squamous cell carcinoma (OSCC) and cervical cancer [5, 7]. Collectively findings from these studies indicate that NDRG2 expression is decreased in most tumors. Moreover, NDRG2 expression was positively correlated with tumor differentiation but negatively correlated with lymph node metastasis and TNM stage (**Figure 1**).

We used a hospital-based study cohort of 226 colorectal cancer patients to analyze the correlation of *NDRG2* mRNA levels with the tumor clinicopathologic features, disease-free survival, and overall survival of colorectal cancer patients. *NDRG2* mRNA expression was significantly correlated with differentiation status, lymph node metastasis, and tumor-node-metastasis stage [23]. Patients with reduced NDRG2 mRNA levels had significantly worse progression-free survival (PFS) and

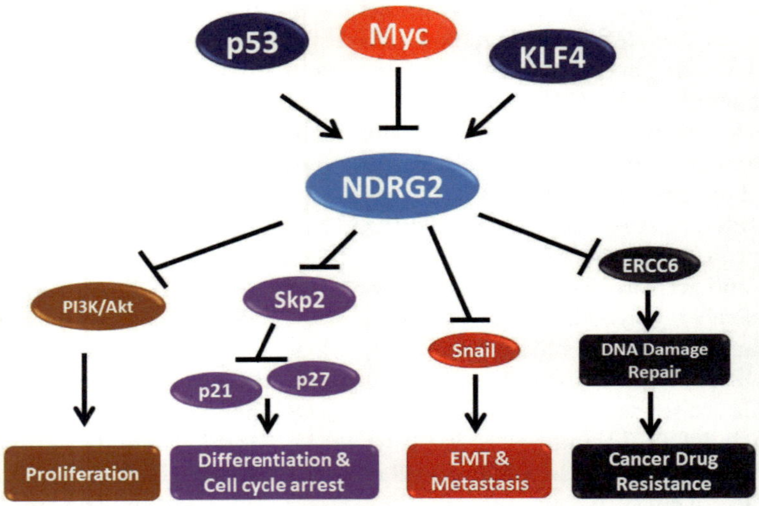

Figure 1.
The molecular working model of NDRG2. NDRG2 can be transcriptionally upregulated by p53 and KLF4, and repressed by Myc. NDRG2 inhibited cancer cells proliferation through blocking PI_3K*/Akt signaling, promoted colorectal cancer cells differentiation through decreasing SKP2 and increasing p21/p27 expression, inhibited EMT through Snail abrogation, and sensitized cancer cells to chemotherapy with DNA damage repair inhibition.*

overall survival (OS) than patients with preserved expression of NDRG2 mRNA. We provided the first evidence that the NDRG2 mRNA level is a novel independent prognostic biomarker for both PFS and OS in colorectal cancer patients [23].

Another study analyzed NDRG2 expression in 127 bladder cancer patients and 97 healthy controls. Similar to the findings in colorectal cancer, NDRG2 expression was significantly downregulated at both the mRNA and protein levels in the urine of patients with bladder cancer and was independently correlated with tumor grade and stage [30]. Thus, NDRG2 expression was decreased in patients with bladder cancer and might be a potential independent diagnostic biomarker for bladder cancer.

5. NDRG2 and differentiation

Differentiation deficiency is a key characteristic of cancer. Poorly differentiated cancers show high proliferation and metastasis capacities, which seriously impact patient survival and prognosis [31]. As a member of the human NDRG gene family, the involvement of NDRG2 in the regulation of cell differentiation has been fully addressed. Bioinformatics analysis of NDRG2 revealed several binding sequences for different transcription factors, which are mostly involved in growth regulation and early differentiation.

As a master switch for cell proliferation and differentiation, Myc performs its biological functions mainly through transcriptional regulation of its target genes, which are involved in cell interaction and communication with their external environment [32, 33]. We first provided the evidence that NDRG2 is transcriptionally repressed by Myc [34]. In addition, c-Myc overexpression dramatically reduced NDRG2 protein and mRNA levels. The core promoter region of NDRG2 is required for Myc-mediated repression of NDRG2 transcription, and the interaction of Myc with the core promoter region was verified both in vitro and in vivo. A mechanistic study showed that Miz-1 is involved in Myc-mediated NDRG2 repression, and is possibly through the recruitment of other epigenetic factors, such as histone deacetylases, to the promoter.

In colorectal cancer, the vast majority of poorly differentiated cells contain constitutive activation of WNT/β-catenin signal. WNT signaling-activating truncation mutations in adenomatous polyposis coli (APC) induce the nuclear translocation of β-catenin is induced, and consequently contributes to cell-fate determination *via* β-catenin/TCF complexes [35–38]. GSK-3β phosphorylates β-catenin at critical serine and threonine residues in its N terminus, which earmarks β-catenin for ubiquitination by the SCF complex and for subsequent degradation by the proteasome pathway [39, 40]. GSK-3β inactivation by APC mutation or oncogenic PI3K/AKT activation leads to the β-catenin/TCF complex formation, and further induced TCF target gene expressions, such as Myc, cyclin D1 [41, 42]. NDRG2 suppresses β-catenin nuclear translocation and decreases the occupancy of β-catenin/TCF complex on the promoter of E3 ligase Skp2, potentially through dephosphorylating AKT and GSK-3β. NDRG2-mediated suppression of Skp2 contributes to the induction and stabilization of p21 and p27, which are target proteins for Skp2-mediated degradation. Thus, NDRG2-meidated induction of cell differentiation is dependent on suppressing the activity of the Skp2 E3 ligase. In support of the biological significance of the reciprocal relationship between NDRG2 and Skp2, an $NDRG2_{low}$/$Skp2_{high}$ gene expression signature correlates with poor patient outcome and could be considered as a diagnostic marker for colorectal cancers.

Additionally, other groups have provided evidence of NDRG2 involvement of cell differentiation induced by different transcription factors, such as Wilms' tumor gene 1 (WT1) protein, HIF-1α and glucocorticoids [33, 54, 55]. Through an oligonucleotide array approach, WT1 was found to indirectly or directly induce the expression of NDRG2 mRNA in CD34+ cells and in leukemic U937 cells through an [54]. Moreover, a novel start site for NDRG2 expression appeared to be used in WT1-transduced cells, suggesting that this promoter is utilized preferentially when high levels of WT1 are present [54].

6. NDRG2 inhibits EMT and cancer metastasis

Metastasis is a unique feature of tumor cells and an important factor affecting the survival and prognosis of cancer patients; it is also an important reason that surgery cannot completely remove tumor lesions. EMT is an important process preceding tumor metastasis [43, 44]. During EMT, tumor cells change from an epithelioid morphology to a mesenchymal cell morphology. The adhesion abilities between cells were decreased [45, 46]. Various signaling pathways were found involved in the regulation of EMT, such as, TGF-β pathway [47], Wnt/β-catenin pathway [48] and Notch pathway [49].

Data indicate that NDRG2 is negatively regulated by TGF-β during the progression of hepatocellular carcinomas [6]. This observation may be due to impairment in the TGF-β/Smad signaling pathway or the activation of non-Smad signaling cascades (PI3K/AKT, p38MAPK and so on) in these cell lines in response to TGF-β. Accordingly, related evidence has shown that the enhancement of GSK-3β activity by NDRG2 overexpression causes proteasomal degradation of the Snail transcription factor and subsequent transcriptional regulation of EMT-related genes [50]. Thus, the tumor suppressor NDRG2 could inhibit TGF-β-induced EMT as well as cell invasion and migration in various cancers. Similarly, a study showed the inhibitory effect of NDRG2 on TGF-β-induced tumor metastasis *via* the attenuation of active autocrine TGF-β production [51].

In breast cancer, NDRG2 downregulated the expression of Snail, as well as the phosphorylation of signal transducer and activator of transcription 3 (STAT3), an oncogenic transcription factor activated in many human malignancies, including breast cancer [24]. Further, NDRG2 overexpressing breast cancer cells showed markedly decreased Snail expression after treatment with STAT3 inhibitors. Thus, the inhibition of STAT3 signaling by NDRG2 suppresses EMT progression *via* the down-regulation of Snail expression. Moreover, high NDRG2 expression induced inactivation of NF-κB and PI3K/AKT signaling pathways *via* the dephosphorylation of the C-terminal domain of PTEN, and the inhibition of the EMT process in OSCC [7]. Therefore, NDRG2 may regulate tumor EMT *via* different regulatory mechanisms in different cancers.

7. NDRG2 is involved in cancer metabolism by regulating glycolysis, glutaminolysis and fatty acid oxidation (FAO)

A cancerous cell undergoes multiple steps to form a solid tumor entity, during which nutrient and oxygen supply insufficiencies frequently occur. In recent decades, studies have provided deep insight into cancer metabolism. In addition to glycolysis, metabolic alterations involve almost all metabolic pathways, including those of lipids, amino acids, nitrogen, and nucleic acids. Metabolic reprogramming is widely accepted to be a hallmark of cancer [52]. Cancer metabolic reprogramming has been further summarized into six hallmarks, including alterations in nutrient uptake (deregulated uptake of glucose and amino acids and the use of opportunistic modes of nutrient acquisition) and intracellular metabolic pathways (the use of glycolysis/TCA cycle intermediates for biosynthesis and NADPH production and an increased demand for nitrogen) [53]. For instance, cancer cells use glucose and glutamine as the major sources of energy and precursor intermediates, thus exhibiting enhanced glycolysis and glutaminolysis [53]. Under various stress conditions, such as, glucose deficiency, cancer cells can shift from glycolysis to FAO to maintain ATP levels and satisfy nutrient demands [54]. Not surprisingly, oncogene activation and tumor suppressor inactivation are extensively involved in these processes. For example, c-Myc, HIF-1α, and p53 can regulate the uptake of both glucose and glutamine and glycolytic flux by affecting the expression of glucose transporters and metabolic enzymes [53].

As a tumor suppressor, NDRG2 was found to regulate aerobic glycolysis and glutaminolysis in cancer cells. A previous study from our laboratory showed that NDRG2 inhibits glucose uptake by interacting with and promoting the degradation of glucose transporter 1 (GLUT1) without affecting its transcription in breast cancer cell lines [55]. Recently, Xu et al. [56] from our laboratory, using colorectal cancer cells and a xenograft model, also demonstrated that NDRG2 inhibits glucose uptake and glycolysis by suppressing the expression and activity of the glucose transporter GLUT1 and key glycolytic enzymes, including hexokinase 2 (HK2), pyruvate kinase M2 isoform (PKM2) and lactate dehydrogenase A (LDHA). In addition, NDRG2 inhibits glutaminolysis by suppressing the expression of the glutamine transporter ASC amino acid transporter 2 (ASCT2) and glutaminase 1 (GLS1) at the transcriptional level. Mechanistically, NDRG2 exerts such effects by suppressing the expression of β-catenin, leading to the repression of its target gene c-Myc. Since c-Myc is a master regulator of metabolism, additional in-depth studies on NDRG2's regulatory role in other tumor glucose catabolism pathways are needed.

Under stress conditions such as glucose limitation, FAO is always activated to preserve the supply of ATP and NADPH [54]. Interestingly, our most recent study [4] revealed that NDRG2, as a negative regulator of AMPK, suppresses glucose deprivation-induced activation of the AMPK/ACC pathway and the consequent induction of FAO genes in hepatoma cells. Thus, NDRG2 overexpression leads to dysregulation of ATP and NADPH, thereby reducing the tolerance of hepatoma cells to glucose limitation. Together, these data further our understanding of the tumor-suppressive mechanism of NDRG2 through its involvement in cancer metabolic reprogramming. Therefore, the application of NDRG2 alone or in combination with antiglycolytic agents such as 2-diacylglycerol (2-DG) may effectively and synergistically inhibit cancer cells, which rely heavily on either glycolysis under non-stressful conditions or FAO under conditions of metabolic stress.

8. NDRG2 knockout enhances tumorigenesis in vivo

Most of the evidence for the role of NDRG2 as a tumor suppressor was mainly obtained in vitro, and establishing an in vivo mouse model to confirm these findings was crucial. It is reported that *Ndrg2*-deficient mice are susceptible to spontaneous tumor formation in vivo and *Ndrg2* knockout mice developed various types of tumors, including lymphomas, hepatocellular carcinomas and bronchoalveolar carcinomas [28]. However, we did not replicate these findings in our established Ndrg2 knockout mouse model—indeed, we did not detect any tumorigenesis in mice at 24 months of age. This discrepancy might be due to the different mouse strains and knockout strategies.

Notably, we established intestine-specific *Ndrg2* knockout mice using a Villin-Cre; *Ndrg2*$^{flox/flox}$ strategy [57]. Intestinal *Ndrg2* deficiency significantly augmented colitis initiation and colitis-associated tumor development. Ndrg2 loss led to the destruction of adherens junction structure *via* E-cadherin reduction, resulting in diminished epithelial barrier function and enhanced gut permeability. We identified the novel mechanism by which NDRG2 is crucial for the interaction of the E3 ligase FBXO11 with Snail, the repressor of E-cadherin. Thus, Ndrg2 loss increased Snail protein stability and decreased E-cadherin expression (https://www.biorxiv.org/content/10.1101/473397v1). Moreover, our study revealed that NDRG2 is an essential intestinal epithelial barrier regulator and plays important roles in gut homeostasis maintenance and colitis-associated tumor development.

Recently, we established a liver cancer metastasis model in WT and Ndrg2 knockout (Ndrg2$^{-/-}$) mice and found that expression loss of the tumor suppressor Ndrg2 in the liver microenvironment significantly suppressed the growth of liver cell colonies [57, 58]. Our data highlighted the role of NDRG2 in the regulation of tumor-associated macrophage (TAM) polarization and its function in promoting cancer liver metastasis. Interestingly, a reduced metastatic burden was correlated with an increased percentage of M1-like TAMs and decreased expression of M2-associated markers in the NDRG2-deficient microenvironment [58]. In summary, our study is the first showing a crucial and unexpected role for NDRG2 in macrophage polarization and highlights the importance of investigating the function of NDRG2 in cancer cells and the tumor microenvironment differently.

9. NDRG2 in brain tumors and other nervous system diseases

Accumulating studies have shown that NDRG2 is associated with various nervous system diseases, including tumors, ischemic stroke, hemorrhage, trauma, and neurodegenerative disorders [1, 59]. NDRG2 was repeatedly reported to be downregulated in a variety of cerebral tumors, including glioma and meningioma [21, 60–66]. The transcription levels of human *NDRG2* are significantly reduced in human glioblastoma tissues and human glioblastoma cell lines, and exogenous overexpression of NDRG2 repressed glioblastoma cell proliferation in vitro [2]. Although direct structural alterations such as point mutations are very rare in the

NDRG2 gene, hypermethylation of the *NDRG2* promoter region was shown to be highly correlated with decreased *NDRG2* transcription levels in human glioblastoma [60, 61, 67, 68]. In addition to the direct impact of *NDRG2* hypermethylation *per se*, NDRG2 may control glioma cell growth by upregulating the levels of histone acetylation in glioma cells [62]. Moreover, the expression level of *NDRG2* was negatively correlated with the pathological grade of the brain tumors and positively correlated with survival in astrocytoma patients [21, 63]. Consistent with the results in glioblastoma, a decrease in the levels of *NDRG2* gene methylation and NDRG2 protein expression were detected in human meningioma [64]. In addition, the expression levels of NDRG2 were significantly further reduced in recurrent meningioma compared to that in primary meningioma [65]. The above results suggest that NDRG2 may be a potential biomarker for predicting the prognosis of human brain tumors.

NDRG family members are abundantly expressed in brain tissue; therefore, the significant functions of these NDRG2 family members in the central nervous system were anticipated and have been confirmed with *NDRG* gene knockout mice-based studies [69–71]. NDRG1 deficiency leads to a progressive demyelinating in the peripheral nerves, suggesting that *NDRG1* is involved in the maintenance of and axonal survival and myelin sheath structure [69]. *Ndrg2*$^{-/-}$ mice exhibited typical ADHD-like behaviors, including hyperactivity, impulsivity, and inattention, as well as impaired memory [70]. *Ndrg4*$^{-/-}$ mice showed impaired cognition and increased susceptibility to ischemic stroke, indicating that NDRG4 has a potential neuroprotective effect [71].

In addition, NDRG2 was implicated in the ischemic stress response in several in vivo and in vitro studies [72–78]. Temporal and spatial patterns of NDRG2 expression in the rat brain were investigated after transient middle cerebral artery occlusion and reperfusion. Both the mRNA and protein levels of NDRG2 were increased following reperfusion in the ischemic penumbra, and NDRG2 was translocated from the cytoplasm to the nucleus in astrocytes. Moreover, NDRG2 expression increased in parallel with the enhancement of TUNEL signals in this ischemic animal model [73]. It is consistent with the results of the animal experiments described above, the expression of NDRG2 was also revealed to be upregulated and NDRG2 can translocate from the cytoplasm to the nucleus in C6-originated astrocytes after oxygen-glucose deprivation (OGD) treatment mimicking ischemic model in vitro [72]. Furthermore, NDRG2 was implicated in some types of cerebral ischemic preconditioning-mediated neuroprotection, including electroacupuncture (EA) [75] and sevoflurane preconditioning [74]. EA preconditioning in the Baihui acupoint was performed before transient focal cerebral ischemia and reperfusion. After EA pretreatment, the number of apoptotic cells in the ischemic penumbra and the volume of cerebral infarct were significantly decreased, and the neurological outcomes were effectively rescued. After ischemia treatment, the levels of NDRG2 expression were largely suppressed in the EA pretreatment group compared with sham group. And NDRG2 was mostly localized in the astroglial cytoplasm; only weak staining was found in the astroglial nucleus after EA pretreatment. However, NDRG2 protein was remarkably transferred from the cytoplasm into the nucleus in the sham group [75]. Recently, NDRG2 was also found to exhibit neuroprotective effects with sevoflurane preconditioning in brain ischemia models both in vivo and in vitro [74]. These results together indicate that NDRG2 takes part in the pathological process of brain ischemia-reperfusion injury and that NDRG2 may be a potential intervention target for ischemic stroke.

NDRG2 has also been repeatedly reported to be associated with other nervous system diseases, such as, neurodegeneration [79–81] and depression [82–84]. NDRG2 has been identified as one of six aberrantly phosphorylated proteins in human brains with frontotemporal lobe degeneration, and an increased phosphospectra of NDRG2 was found in these neurodegenerative tissues [85]. Accumulated NDRG2 and GFAP were detected in cortical senile plaques from the postmortem human brain tissues with Alzheimer's disease (AD) [79]. In addition, the expression levels of NDRG2 and GFAP were parallelly increased in amyloid precursor protein (APP)/presenilin (PS1) mouse, a double transgenic AD mouse model [80]. Suppressed NDRG2 expression and decreased memory impairment were detected in parallel after EA treatment to APP/PS1 transgenic mice. Furthermore, the increased reactive astrocytes andNDRG2 expression were detected in the mice which were exposed to 1-methyl-4-phenyl-1,2,3,6-tetrahydropyridine, a Parkinson's disease-associated neurotoxin that causes both glial activation and neurodegeneration [86]. Moreover, growing studies have demonstrated that NDRG2 is related with the function of antidepressants, which can correct depression-like behaviors and alleviate neural damages observed in depressive animals [82–84]. NDRG2 was downregulated in the rat frontal cortex after chronic use of antidepressants [84]. In contrast to the results described above antidepressants did not counteract the increase in NDRG2 expression in the hippocampus of rats with stress-induced depression-like symptoms and that antidepressants *per se* induced NDRG2 expression in normal rats [83]. Further study of the detailed mechanisms by which NDRG2 participates in these neurodegenerative or chronic psychiatric diseases providing novel intervention strategies will thus be interesting.

10. Conclusion and perspectives

To date, both in vitro and in vivo evidence has shown that NDRG2 can inhibit cancer cell proliferation, EMT, metastasis and can promote cell differentiation and cell cycle arrest. Thus, NDRG2 might be a target for cancer treatment and therapeutic resistance. Although NDRG2 is a novel tumor suppressor, the detailed mechanism by which NDRG2 functions requires further elucidation. Moreover, additional in vivo data are needed to confirm its tumor suppressor function.

Author details

Jian Zhang*, Xia Li, Liangliang Shen, Yan Li and Libo Yao
The State Key Laboratory of Cancer Biology, Department of Biochemistry and Molecular Biology, The Fourth Military Medical University, Xian, China

*Address all correspondence to: biozhangj@fmmu.edu.cn

References

[1] Yao L, Zhang J, Liu X. NDRG2: A myc-repressed gene involved in cancer and cell stress. Acta Biochimica et Biophysica Sinica. 2008;**40**:625-635

[2] Deng Y, Yao L, Chau L, Ng SS, Peng Y, Liu X, et al. N-Myc downstream-regulated gene 2 (NDRG2) inhibits glioblastoma cell proliferation. International Journal of Cancer. 2003;**106**:342-347

[3] Liu N, Wang L, Liu X, Yang Q, Zhang J, Zhang W, et al. Promoter methylation, mutation, and genomic deletion are involved in the decreased NDRG2 expression levels in several cancer cell lines. Biochemical and Biophysical Research Communications. 2007;**358**:164-169

[4] Pan T, Zhang M, Zhang F, Yan G, Ru Y, Wang Q, et al. NDRG2 overexpression suppresses hepatoma cells survival during metabolic stress through disturbing the activation of fatty acid oxidation. Biochemical and Biophysical Research Communications. 2017;**483**:860-866

[5] Liu J, Yang L, Zhang J, Zhang J, Chen Y, Li K, et al. Knock-down of NDRG2 sensitizes cervical cancer Hela cells to cisplatin through suppressing Bcl-2 expression. BMC Cancer. 2012;**12**:370

[6] Lee DC, Kang YK, Kim WH, Jang YJ, Kim DJ, Park IY, et al. Functional and clinical evidence for NDRG2 as a candidate suppressor of liver cancer metastasis. Cancer Research. 2008;**68**:4210-4220

[7] Tamura T, Ichikawa T, Nakahata S, Kondo Y, Tagawa Y, Yamamoto K, et al. Loss of NDRG2 expression confers oral squamous cell carcinoma with enhanced metastatic potential. Cancer Research. 2017;**77**: 2363-2374

[8] Shen L, Qu X, Li H, Xu C, Wei M, Wang Q, et al. NDRG2 facilitates colorectal cancer differentiation through the regulation of Skp2-p21/p27 axis. Oncogene. 2018;**37**:1759-1774

[9] Wang L, Liu N, Yao L, Li F, Zhang J, Deng Y, et al. NDRG2 is a new HIF-1 target gene necessary for hypoxia-induced apoptosis in A549 cells. Cellular Physiology and Biochemistry. 2008;**21**:239-250

[10] Cao W, Zhang JL, Feng DY, Liu XW, Li Y, Wang LF, et al. The effect of adenovirus-conjugated NDRG2 on p53-mediated apoptosis of hepatocarcinoma cells through attenuation of nucleotide excision repair capacity. Biomaterials. 2014;**35**:993-1003

[11] Liu N, Wang L, Li X, Yang Q, Liu X, Zhang J, et al. N-myc downstream-regulated gene 2 is involved in p53-mediated apoptosis. Nucleic Acids Research. 2008;**36**:5335-5349

[12] Wei Y, Yu S, Zhang Y, Zhang Y, Zhao H, Xiao Z, et al. NDRG2 promotes adriamycin sensitivity through a Bad/p53 complex at the mitochondria in breast cancer. Oncotarget. 2017;**8**:29038-29047

[13] Hetz C. The unfolded protein response: Controlling cell fate decisions under ER stress and beyond. Nature Reviews. Molecular Cell Biology. 2012;**13**:89-102

[14] Hetz C, Chevet E, Harding HP. Targeting the unfolded protein response in disease. Nature Reviews. Drug Discovery. 2013;**12**:703-719

[15] Cao SS, Kaufman RJ. Unfolded protein response. Current Biology. 2012;**22**:R622-R626

[16] Wang M, Kaufman RJ. The impact of the endoplasmic reticulum

protein-folding environment on cancer development. Nature Reviews. Cancer. 2014;**14**:581-597

[17] Zhang M, Liu X, Wang Q, Ru Y, Xiong X, Wu K, et al. NDRG2 acts as a PERK co-factor to facilitate PERK branch and ERS-induced cell death. FEBS Letters. 2017;**591**:3670-3681

[18] Hu XL, Liu XP, Deng YC, Lin SX, Wu L, Zhang J, et al. Expression analysis of the NDRG2 gene in mouse embryonic and adult tissues. Cell and Tissue Research. 2006;**325**:67-76

[19] Shen L, Zhao ZY, Wang YZ, Ji SP, Liu XP, Liu XW, et al. Immunohistochemical detection of Ndrg2 in the mouse nervous system. Neuroreport. 2008;**19**:927-931

[20] Hou WG, Zhao Y, Shen L, Zhao J, Liu XW, Li Z, et al. Differential expression of N-Myc downstream regulated gene 2 (NDRG2) in the rat testis during postnatal development. Cell and Tissue Research. 2009;**337**:257-267

[21] Li W, Chu D, Chu X, Meng F, Wei D, Li H, et al. Decreased expression of NDRG2 is related to poor overall survival in patients with glioma. Journal of Clinical Neuroscience: Official Journal of the Neurosurgical Society of Australasia. 2011;**18**:1534-1537

[22] Shen L, Qu X, Ma Y, Zheng J, Chu D, Liu B, et al. Tumor suppressor NDRG2 tips the balance of oncogenic TGF-β via EMT inhibition in colorectal cancer. Oncogene. 2014;**3**:e86. DOI: 10.1038/oncsis.2013.48

[23] Chu D, Zhang Z, Li Y, Wu L, Zhang J, Wang W, et al. Prediction of colorectal cancer relapse and prognosis by tissue mRNA levels of NDRG2. Molecular Cancer Therapeutics. 2011;**10**:47-56

[24] Kim MJ, Lim J, Yang Y, Lee MS, Lim JS. N-myc downstream-regulated gene 2 (NDRG2) suppresses the epithelial-mesenchymal transition (EMT) in breast cancer cells *via* STAT3/Snail signaling. Cancer Letters. 2014;**354**:33-42

[25] Tantai J, Pan X, Hu D. RNF4-mediated SUMOylation is essential for NDRG2 suppression of lung adenocarcinoma. Oncotarget. 2016;**7**:26837-26843

[26] Mordalska A, Latek J, Ferenc T, Pomorski L, Galecka E, Zygmunt A, et al. Evaluation of NDRG2 gene expression in primary papillary thyroid carcinoma and in metastases of this neoplasm to regional lymph nodes. Thyroid Research. 2010;**3**:6

[27] Zhao H, Zhang J, Lu J, He X, Chen C, Li X, et al. Reduced expression of N-Myc downstream-regulated gene 2 in human thyroid cancer. BMC Cancer. 2008;**8**:303

[28] Nakahata S, Ichikawa T, Maneesaay P, Saito Y, Nagai K, Tamura T, et al. Loss of NDRG2 expression activates PI3K-AKT signalling *via* PTEN phosphorylation in ATLL and other cancers. Nature Communications. 2014;**5**:3393

[29] Tschan MP, Shan D, Laedrach J, Eyholzer M, Leibundgut EO, Baerlocher GM, et al. NDRG1/2 expression is inhibited in primary acute myeloid leukemia. Leukemia Research. 2010;**34**:393-398

[30] Zhang M, Ren B, Li Z, Niu W, Wang Y. Expression of N-myc downstream-regulated gene 2 in bladder cancer and its potential utility as a urinary diagnostic biomarker. Medical Science Monitor. 2017;**23**:4644-4649

[31] Derwinger K, Kodeda K, Bexe-Lindskog E, Taflin H. Tumour differentiation grade is associated with TNM staging and the risk of node metastasis in colorectal cancer. Acta Oncologica. 2010;**49**:57-62

[32] Vervoorts J, Luscher-Firzlaff J, Luscher B. The ins and outs of MYC regulation by posttranslational mechanisms. The Journal of Biological Chemistry. 2006;**281**:34725-34729

[33] Grandori C, Cowley SM, James LP, Eisenman RN. The Myc/Max/Mad network and the transcriptional control of cell behavior. Annual Review of Cell and Developmental Biology. 2000;**16**:653-699

[34] Zhang J, Li F, Liu X, Shen L, Liu J, Su J, et al. The repression of human differentiation-related gene NDRG2 expression by Myc *via* Miz-1-dependent interaction with the NDRG2 core promoter. The Journal of Biological Chemistry. 2006;**281**:39159-39168

[35] Goss KH, Groden J. Biology of the adenomatous polyposis coli tumor suppressor. Journal of Clinical Oncology: Official Journal of the American Society of Clinical Oncology. 2000;**18**:1967-1979

[36] Morin PJ, Sparks AB, Korinek V, Barker N, Clevers H, Vogelstein B, et al. Activation of beta-catenin-Tcf signaling in colon cancer by mutations in beta-catenin or APC. Science. 1997;**275**:1787-1790

[37] Bienz M, Clevers H. Linking colorectal cancer to Wnt signaling. Cell. 2000;**103**:311-320

[38] Ng RC, Matsumaru D, Ho AS, Garcia-Barcelo MM, Yuan ZW, Smith D, et al. Dysregulation of Wnt inhibitory factor 1 (Wif1) expression resulted in aberrant Wnt-beta-catenin signaling and cell death of the cloaca endoderm, and anorectal malformations. Cell Death and Differentiation. 2014;**21**:978-989

[39] Aberle H, Bauer A, Stappert J, Kispert A, Kemler R. Beta-catenin is a target for the ubiquitin-proteasome pathway. The EMBO Journal. 1997;**16**:3797-3804

[40] Marikawa Y, Elinson RP. Beta-TrCP is a negative regulator of Wnt/beta-catenin signaling pathway and dorsal axis formation in *Xenopus* embryos. Mechanisms of Development. 1998;**77**:75-80

[41] He TC, Sparks AB, Rago C, Hermeking H, Zawel L, da Costa LT, et al. Identification of c-MYC as a target of the APC pathway. Science. 1998;**281**:1509-1512

[42] Tetsu O, McCormick F. Beta-catenin regulates expression of cyclin D1 in colon carcinoma cells. Nature. 1999;**398**:422-426

[43] Hugo H, Ackland ML, Blick T, Lawrence MG, Clements JA, Williams ED, et al. Epithelial-mesenchymal and mesenchymal-epithelial transitions in carcinoma progression. Journal of Cellular Physiology. 2007;**213**:374-383

[44] Foroni C, Broggini M, Generali D, Damia G. Epithelial-mesenchymal transition and breast cancer: Role, molecular mechanisms and clinical impact. Cancer Treatment Reviews. 2012;**38**:689-697

[45] Boyer B, Valles AM, Edme N. Induction and regulation of epithelial-mesenchymal transitions. Biochemical Pharmacology. 2000;**60**:1091-1099

[46] Thiery JP. Epithelial-mesenchymal transitions in tumour progression. Nature Reviews. Cancer. 2002;**2**:442-454

[47] Saitoh M, Miyazawa K. Transcriptional and post-transcriptional regulation in TGF-beta-mediated epithelial-mesenchymal transition. Journal of Biochemistry. 2012;**151**:563-571

[48] Gilles C, Polette M, Mestdagt M, Nawrocki-Raby B, Ruggeri P, Birembaut P, et al. Transactivation of vimentin by beta-catenin in human breast cancer cells. Cancer Research. 2003;**63**:2658-2664

[49] Wang Z, Li Y, Kong D, Sarkar FH. The role of Notch signaling pathway in epithelial-mesenchymal transition (EMT) during development and tumor aggressiveness. Current Drug Targets. 2010;**11**:745-751

[50] Kim YJ, Kang HB, Yim HS, Kim JH, Kim JW. NDRG2 positively regulates E-cadherin expression and prolongs overall survival in colon cancer patients. Oncology Reports. 2013;**30**:1890-1898

[51] Oh SS, Kim D, Kim DH, Chang HH, Sohn KC, Kim KH, et al. NDRG2 correlated with favorable recurrence-free survival inhibits metastasis of mouse breast cancer cells *via* attenuation of active TGF-beta production. Carcinogenesis. 2012;**33**:1882-1888

[52] Hanahan D, Weinberg RA. Hallmarks of cancer: The next generation. Cell. 2011;**144**:646-674

[53] Pavlova NN, Thompson CB. The emerging hallmarks of cancer metabolism. Cell Metabolism. 2016;**23**:27-47

[54] Carracedo A, Cantley LC, Pandolfi PP. Cancer metabolism: Fatty acid oxidation in the limelight. Nature Reviews. Cancer. 2013;**13**:227-232

[55] Vriend J, Reiter RJ. The Keap1-Nrf2-antioxidant response element pathway: A review of its regulation by melatonin and the proteasome. Molecular and Cellular Endocrinology. 2015;**401**:213-220

[56] Xu X, Li J, Sun X, Guo Y, Chu D, Wei L, et al. Tumor suppressor NDRG2 inhibits glycolysis and glutaminolysis in colorectal cancer cells by repressing c-Myc expression. Oncotarget. 2015;**6**:26161-26176

[57] von Karstedt S. NDRG2 programs tumor-associated macrophages for tumor support. Cell Death & Disease. 2018;**9**:294

[58] Li M, Lai X, Zhao Y, Zhang Y, Li M, Li D, et al. Loss of NDRG2 in liver microenvironment inhibits cancer liver metastasis by regulating tumor associate macrophages polarization. Cell Death & Disease. 2018;**9**:248

[59] Lin K, Yin A, Yao L, Li Y. N-myc downstream-regulated gene 2 in the nervous system: From expression pattern to function. Acta Biochimica et Biophysica Sinica. 2015;**47**:761-766

[60] Zhou B, Tang Z, Deng Y, Hou S, Liu N, Lin W, et al. Tumor suppressor candidate gene, NDRG2 is frequently inactivated in human glioblastoma multiforme. Molecular Medicine Reports. 2014;**10**:891-896

[61] Tepel M, Roerig P, Wolter M, Gutmann DH, Perry A, Reifenberger G, et al. Frequent promoter hypermethylation and transcriptional downregulation of the NDRG2 gene at 14q11.2 in primary glioblastoma. International Journal of Cancer. 2008;**123**:2080-2086

[62] Li L, Qin X, Shi M, Miao R, Wang L, Liu X, et al. Regulation of histone acetylation by NDRG2 in glioma cells. Journal of Neuro-Oncology. 2012;**106**:485-492

[63] Li L, Wang J, Shen X, Wang L, Li X, Liu Y, et al. Expression and prognostic value of NDRG2 in human astrocytomas. Journal of the Neurological Sciences. 2011;**308**:77-82

[64] Lusis EA, Watson MA, Chicoine MR, Lyman M, Roerig P, Reifenberger G, et al. Integrative genomic analysis

identifies NDRG2 as a candidate tumor suppressor gene frequently inactivated in clinically aggressive meningioma. Cancer Research. 2005;**65**:7121-7126

[65] Skiriute D, Tamasauskas S, Asmoniene V, Saferis V, Skauminas K, Deltuva V, et al. Tumor grade-related NDRG2 gene expression in primary and recurrent intracranial meningiomas. Journal of Neuro-Oncology. 2011;**102**:89-94

[66] Zhang ZG, Li G, Feng DY, Zhang J, Zhang J, Qin HZ, et al. Overexpression of NDRG2 can inhibit neuroblastoma cell proliferation through negative regulation by CYR61. Asian Pacific Journal of Cancer Prevention: APJCP. 2014;**15**:239-244

[67] Skiriute D, Vaitkiene P, Asmoniene V, Steponaitis G, Deltuva VP, Tamasauskas A. Promoter methylation of AREG, HOXA11, hMLH1, NDRG2, NPTX2 and Tes genes in glioblastoma. Journal of Neuro-Oncology. 2013;**113**:441-449

[68] Skiriute D, Steponaitis G, Vaitkiene P, Mikuciunas M, Skauminas K, Tamasauskas A, et al. Glioma malignancy-dependent NDRG2 gene methylation and downregulation correlates with poor patient outcome. Journal of Cancer. 2014;**5**:446-456

[69] Okuda T, Higashi Y, Kokame K, Tanaka C, Kondoh H, Miyata T. Ndrg1-deficient mice exhibit a progressive demyelinating disorder of peripheral nerves. Molecular and Cellular Biology. 2004;**24**:3949-3956

[70] Li Y, Yin A, Sun X, Zhang M, Zhang J, Wang P, et al. Deficiency of tumor suppressor NDRG2 leads to attention deficit and hyperactive behavior. The Journal of Clinical Investigation. 2017;**127**:4270-4284

[71] Yamamoto H, Kokame K, Okuda T, Nakajo Y, Yanamoto H, Miyata T. NDRG4 protein-deficient mice exhibit spatial learning deficits and vulnerabilities to cerebral ischemia. The Journal of Biological Chemistry. 2011;**286**:26158-26165

[72] Li Y, Xu N, Cai L, Gao Z, Shen L, Zhang Q, et al. NDRG2 is a novel p53-associated regulator of apoptosis in C6-originated astrocytes exposed to oxygen-glucose deprivation. PLoS One. 2013;**8**:e57130

[73] Li Y, Shen L, Cai L, Wang Q, Hou W, Wang F, et al. Spatial-temporal expression of NDRG2 in rat brain after focal cerebral ischemia and reperfusion. Brain Research. 2011;**1382**:252-258

[74] Li X, Luo P, Wang F, Yang Q, Li Y, Zhao M, et al. Inhibition of N-myc downstream-regulated gene-2 is involved in an astrocyte-specific neuroprotection induced by sevoflurane preconditioning. Anesthesiology. 2014;**121**:549-562

[75] Wang F, Gao Z, Li X, Li Y, Li X, Zhong H, et al. NDRG2 is involved in anti-apoptosis induced by electroacupuncture pretreatment after focal cerebral ischemia in rats. Neurological Research. 2013;**35**:406-414

[76] Feng T, Han BH, Yang GL, Shi CJ, Gao ZW, Cao MZ, et al. Neuroprotective influence of miR-301a inhibition in experimental cerebral ischemia/reperfusion rat models through targeting NDRG2. Journal of Molecular Neuroscience. May 2019;**68**(1):144-152

[77] Ma YL, Zhang LX, Liu GL, Fan Y, Peng Y, Hou WG. N-myc downstream-regulated gene 2 (Ndrg2) is involved in ischemia-hypoxia-induced astrocyte apoptosis: A novel target for stroke therapy. Molecular Neurobiology. 2017;**54**:3286-3299

[78] Takarada-Iemata M, Yoshikawa A, Ta HM, Okitani N, Nishiuchi T, Aida Y, et al. N-myc downstream-regulated

gene 2 protects blood-brain barrier integrity following cerebral ischemia. Glia. 2018;**66**:1432-1446

[79] Mitchelmore C, Buchmann-Moller S, Rask L, West MJ, Troncoso JC, Jensen NA. NDRG2: A novel Alzheimer's disease associated protein. Neurobiology of Disease. 2004;**16**:48-58

[80] Wang F, Zhong H, Li X, Peng Y, Kinden R, Liang W, et al. Electroacupuncture attenuates reference memory impairment associated with astrocytic NDRG2 suppression in APP/PS1 transgenic mice. Molecular Neurobiology. 2014;**50**:305-313

[81] Rong XF, Sun YN, Liu DM, Yin HJ, Peng Y, Xu SF, et al. The pathological roles of NDRG2 in Alzheimer's disease, a study using animal models and APPwt-overexpressed cells. CNS Neuroscience & Therapeutics. 2017;**23**:667-679

[82] Nichols NR. Ndrg2, a novel gene regulated by adrenal steroids and antidepressants, is highly expressed in astrocytes. Annals of the New York Academy of Sciences. 2003;**1007**:349-356

[83] Araya-Callis C, Hiemke C, Abumaria N, Flugge G. Chronic psychosocial stress and citalopram modulate the expression of the glial proteins GFAP and NDRG2 in the hippocampus. Psychopharmacology. 2012;**224**:209-222

[84] Takahashi K, Yamada M, Ohata H, Momose K, Higuchi T, Honda K, et al. Expression of Ndrg2 in the rat frontal cortex after antidepressant and electroconvulsive treatment. The International Journal of Neuropsychopharmacology. 2005;**8**:381-389

[85] Herskowitz JH, Seyfried NT, Duong DM, Xia Q, Rees HD, Gearing M, et al. Phosphoproteomic analysis reveals site-specific changes in GFAP and NDRG2 phosphorylation in frontotemporal lobar degeneration. Journal of Proteome Research. 2010;**9**:6368-6379

[86] Takeichi T, Takarada-Iemata M, Hashida K, Sudo H, Okuda T, Kokame K, et al. The effect of Ndrg2 expression on astroglial activation. Neurochemistry International. 2011;**59**:21-27

Chapter 2

METCAM/MUC18: A Novel Tumor Suppressor for Some Cancers

Guang-Jer Wu

Abstract

METCAM/MUC18, a component of cellular membrane, is a cell adhesion molecule (CAM) in the Ig-like gene super-family. It is capable of carrying out general functions of CAMs, such as performing intercellular interactions and interaction of cell with extracellular matrix in tumor microenvironment, interacting with various signaling pathways, and regulating social behaviors of cells. METCAM/MUC18 plays the tumor suppressor function in some cancers, such as colorectal cancer, nasopharyngeal carcinoma type I, one mouse melanoma subline K1735-9, ovarian cancer, pancreatic cancer, prostate cancer PC-3 cell line, and perhaps hemangioma. Possible mechanism in the METCAM/MUC18-mediated tumor suppression is proposed. By taking advantage of the tumor suppressor function of METCAM/MUC18, recombinant METCAM/MUC18 proteins and other derived products may be used as therapeutic agents to treat these cancers.

Keywords: METCAM/MUC18, Ig-like CAM, *in vivo* tumor suppression, colorectal cancer, nasopharyngeal carcinoma, mouse melanoma, ovarian cancer, pancreatic cancer, prostate cancer, mouse models

1. Introduction: tumor initiation and malignant progression is mainly controlled by two sets of genes as well as CAMs

Tumor/cancer is a genetic disease due to accumulated mutations or epigenetic alterations in our genetic material, DNA [1]. 80–90% of cancer risk comes from environmental factors and the remaining 10–20% risk from hereditary factors [2]. Environment in a broad sense includes both the physical containment and the social and cultural environment and its associated effects on our lifestyle choices. The environmental factors in the physical containment include chemicals (from polluted drinking water, air and soil, and diet), physical agents (UV and environmental radiation and medical radiation), biological agents (tumor viruses, bacteria, and parasites), and the lifestyle. These agents aim to attack our DNA in the somatic cells and resulting in accumulation of mutations and epigenetic alterations in our genes throughout our life time. Hereditary factors (lineage specific cues) include both the inherited genetic mutations and epigenetic imprinting in the germ cells that pass on from generation to generation. Tumor initiation and malignant progression are mainly caused by two sets of genes, such as the tumor-promoting genes (oncogenes) and the tumor suppressor genes, thus, mutations and epigenetic alterations in these two sets of genes are doom to be responsible for the tumorigenic process [2–4].

In addition to exogenous chemical agents, physical agents, and biological agents in the environment that cause mutations in the genes, endogenous metabolic processes and chronic inflammation from our lifestyle choices produce free radicals that directly attack our DNA also resulting in mutations [5]. The major sources of free radicals are reactive oxygen species (ROS), which is a collective term for the unstable, reactive, partially reduced oxygen derivatives that are the normal by-products of our metabolic processes. They include hydrogen peroxide (H_2O_2), superoxide anion (O_2^-), hypochlorous acid (HOCl), singlet oxygen ($^1O_2$), and hydroxyl radical ($^{\bullet}HO$). ROS are also produced by the inflammatory macrophages and neutrophils and are spilled out to attack the DNA of bystander cells. ROS acts as the secondary messengers in cell signaling and essential for various biological processes in both normal and cancer cells and as both tumor-promoting and tumor suppressing agents. To keep the system in check, ROS is balanced by intracellular anti-oxidant enzymes, that produce a number of anti-oxidants, such as glutathione (GSH) and thioredoxin (Txn), which are also present in our foodstuffs, to remove ROS. ROS production is a mechanism shared by most chemotherapeutics to trigger cell-death in cancer cells and unfortunately also to some extent in normal cells. Thus, ROS has conflicting roles as a secondary messenger in cancer cells as well as cancer-killers during cancer chemotherapy.

Most of the mutations in the oncogenes are dominant and thus manifest obvious phenotypes of increased proliferation and survival of tumor cells (gain-of-functions). In contrast, most of mutations in the tumor suppressor genes are recessive and thus do not manifest any phenotype until both copies of the gene are mutated or altered epigenetically (loss-of-functions). Some tumor suppressor genes are gate-keepers that directly affect proliferation and death, thus directly open to tumor formation. But some tumor suppressor genes are care-takers that affect DNA repair functions and genomic stability, thus increase mutation rate of all genes and indirectly affect proliferation [2, 6].

Epigenetic alterations may change the extent of methylation (either hypo- or hyper-methylation) in the regulatory regions of both oncogenes and tumor-suppressor genes, thus affect the transcriptionally regulatory region of the genes and directly regulate transcriptional expression of the genes. Epigenetic alterations may also modify histones and non-histone proteins that affect chromosome remodeling, thus indirectly affect the transcription of the genes. Epigenetic alterations may also affect post-transcription processes (namely translational process or stability of mRNA) of the genes via microRNAs [7].

Besides the above traditional two sets of genes, other genes, such as CAMs, also contribute directly to the tumor initiation and progression or orchestrate the tumor microenvironment to affect the tumor progression [8]. CAMs are involved in several biological functions, such as tissue architecture, organ formation, blood vessel generation and angiogenesis, immune and inflammatory reactions, wound healing and social behaviors [8]. An altered expression of CAMs may have implications in tumorigenesis, since CAMs govern cellular social behaviors by directly contributing to cell adhesion and cross-talk with the intracellular signal transduction pathways [8]. As a consequence, an aberrant expression of CAMs is capable of changing mobility and invasiveness, influencing outlasting ability and proliferation of tumor cells, and altering new blood vessel formation [8]. It also affects distant organ-dissemination of carcinoma cells, because CAMs orchestrate complex interactions of tumor cells with various stromal cells in the tumor microenvironment, resulting in augmentation or reduction of the spreading potential of carcinoma cells [8]. Effects of the aberrant expression of the following CAMs on tumorigenesis and malignant progression are better studied, such as cadherin [9], integrins [10], CD44 [11], CEACAM [12], mucins [13], L1CAM [14], EpCAM [15], ALCAM [16] and METCAM/MUC18 [17]. Over the past several years, our team investigated the role of METCAM/MUC18 in several types of tumors, such as melanoma, breast, nasopharyngeal, ovarian and prostate cancers [18–36]. The resulting data showed a dual role of METCAM/MUC18 as a tumor promotor or suppressor in these cancers [17, 37].

2. METCAM/MUC18: an immunoglobulin-like (Ig-like) CAM

Originally, METCAM/MUC18 was first demonstrated to be abundantly expressed on the cellular membrane of most malignant human melanomas, hence named as MUC18. It has been implicated to play a pivotal role in the malignant progression of human melanoma, hence was named as MCAM and Mel-CAM) [38]. However, METCAM/MUC18 was found in subsequent studies not to be exclusively expressed in melanoma, and it did not initiate the transformation of normal cutaneous melanocytes to melanoma either [39]. Instead, METCAM/MUC18 was also expressed in other epithelial tumors and it could initiate or promote the transformation of other epithelial cells into carcinomas [40]. Thus, METCAM/MUC18 also bears other names, such as S-endo1, CD146, A32, or METCAM [40, 41]. Later METCAM/MUC18 was found to be able to suppress tumorigenesis in some cancer cell lines [17, 37, 40].

The human METCAM/MUC18 is a *c*ell *a*dhesion *m*olecule (CAM) belonging to the Ig-like gene superfamily. The naked human METCAM/MUC18 is a single chain transmembrane protein of 65–72 kDa consisting in 646 amino acids with an extracellular N-terminal domain of 558 amino acids, a 24 amino acids-transmembrane domain and a cytoplasmic domain of 64 residues (**Figure 1**) [38, 42].

Figure 1 shows that the N-terminal extra-cellular domain of the protein is composed of a signal peptide sequence (SP) and five immunoglobulin-like domains and one X domain [37, 42]. The intracellular cytoplasmic domain has one, three, and one protein kinase consent sequences that are potentially to be phosphorylated by PKA, PKC, and CK2, respectively [37, 38, 42]. In addition, the METCAM/MUC18 usually has an apparent molecular weight of 110–150,000 because it is heavily glycosylated in all cell types. The amino acid sequence of huMETCAM/MUC18 reveals nine possible N-glycosylation sites, of which six are conserved between human and mouse proteins, in the extracellular domain. METCAM/MUC18 is conserved in mouse, in which the amino acid sequences of mouse METCAM/MUC18 (moMETCAM/MUC18) are 72.6% identical to the huMETCAM/MUC18 [43]. Therefore, both human and mouse METCAM/MUC18's are capable of performing similar general functions of CAMs, such as controlling cellular social behaviors by impacting the adhesion status of cells and modulating signaling. Furthermore, over-expression of both human and mouse METCAM/MUC18's similarly affected tumor cells in *in vitro* motility and invasiveness, *in vitro* and *in vivo* tumorigenesis, and *in vivo* metastasis [42, 43].

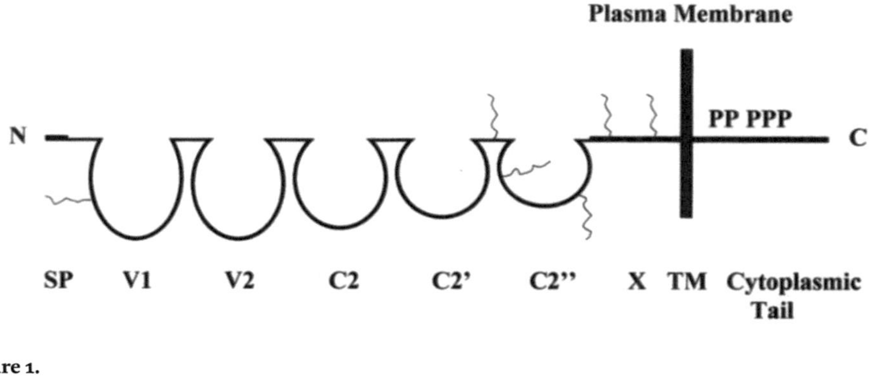

Figure 1.
The human METCAM/MUC18 (huMETCAM/MUC18). The figure represents the protein structure of huMETCAM/MUC18 with its 3 domains: (1) a large extracellular domain showing a signal peptide (SP), the five Ig-like variables (V1 and V2) and conserved (C1, C2, C2' and C2") domains, each of which held together by a disulfide bond, and one X domain; six conserved N-glycosylation sites indicated as wavy lines in V1, the interdomain C2'/C2", C2" and X domains; (2) a short transmembrane domain (TM); and (3) a cytoplasmic domain containing five potential phosphorylation sites (P).

The huMETCAM/MUC18 is expressed in at least 10 normal tissues: hair follicular cells, smooth muscle cells, endothelial cells, cerebellum, basal cells of the lung, activated T cells, intermediate trophoblasts [44], breast epithelium [18, 19], nasopharyngeal epithelium [23], and ovarian epithelium [27]. The protein is also expressed in several carcinomas, such as breast carcinoma, intermediate trophoblast tumors, melanoma, prostate adenocarcinoma, osteosarcoma, and others [17, 44]. Our studies also indicate that over-expression of METCAM/MUC18 augments tumorigenesis of breast carcinoma [18–20], nasopharyngeal carcinoma type III [24, 26], and prostate adenocarcinoma [34], but it does not have an obvious effect on tumorigenesis of most melanoma cell lines [21]. METCAM/MUC18 over-expression also initiates the distant organ-dissemination of prostate cancer [32, 33] and augments the distant organ-dissemination of melanoma [21] and breast carcinoma [45].

In contrast, over-expression of METCAM/MUC18 represses tumorigenesis of a mouse melanoma cell line, K1735-9 [22], nasopharyngeal carcinoma type I [24, 25] and perhaps hemangiomas [46]. METCAM/MUC18 over-expression also represses the distant organ-dissemination of the mouse melanoma cell line, K1735-9 [22].

3. METCAM/MUC18: a tumor suppressor in several types of cancer

3.1 Mouse melanoma

Over-expression of moMETCAM/MUC18 in one mouse melanoma cell line K1735 clone 10 (or K1735-10 subline) has no effect and that in another cell line K1735 clone 3 a slight suppression effect on subcutaneous tumorigenesis [21], but in K1735 clone 9 (or K1735-9 subline) it completely suppresses the subcutaneous tumorigenesis [22]. Thus, METCAM/MUC18 definitely acts as a tumor suppressor for the K1735-9 subline, but may have a less obvious effect on two other K1735 sublines, K1735-3 and K1735-10. In addition to its effect on tumorigenesis, over-expression of moMETCAM/MUC18 in K1735-9 also completely suppressed lung nodule formation in immunocompetent syngeneic C3H brown mouse model. In contrast, over-expression of moMETCAM/MUC18 in K1735-3 and K1735-10 subline has an opposite effect (namely promotion) on lung nodule formation. In conclusion, moMETCAM/MUC18 acts as a tumor suppressor with a different severity on different cell lines in a syngenetic mouse model [21, 22].

3.2 Nasopharyngeal carcinoma

Nasopharyngeal carcinoma (NPC) occurs in the non-lymphomatous, squamous epithelial lining of the posterior nasopharynx [24]. Histologically, three subtypes of NPC are defined according to World Health Organization (WHO) classification: WHO type I (keratinizing squamous cell carcinomas), WHO type II (non-keratinizing squamous cell carcinomas), and WHO type III (undifferentiated carcinomas) [24]. Three major risk factors suggested by epidemiological studies, such as genetic predisposition, dietary and environmental factors, and the Epstein Barr virus (EBV) infection, may cause the unusual occurrence of NPC in endemic areas [24–26]. However, the biological mechanisms of their involvement in cancer initiation, development or malignant progression are not well understood. Nevertheless, it could be hypothesized that altered cell adhesion molecules (CAMs) in NPC lead to tumorigenesis and malignant progression, since aberrant expression of CAMs, such as CD44, connexin 43, E-cadherin, and ICAM, has been associated with the progression of NPC [23]. In order to test this hypothesis, we previously studied the possible role of altered METCAM/MUC18 expression in nasopharyngeal carcinoma [23, 24].

Therefore, we used immunohistochemistry method to determine gene expression at the protein level in seven tissue specimens of normal nasopharynx, 97 specimens of three different types of NPC and also used immunoblot method to determine that in several cell lines established from type I and type III NPC [23]. The results showed a weak expression of the protein METCAM/MUC18 in 27% of the NPC tissues in contrast to all the normal nasopharynx tissues which exhibited high expression of the protein. According to these results, we suggested that METCAM/MUC18 may play a tumor suppressor function in the development of NPC during the progression of the disease [23]. We then tested the hypothesis by transfecting the cDNA into two NPC cell lines which weakly expressed the protein and isolated the high-expressing clones for examining the effect of METCAM/MUC18 over-expression on *in vitro* cellular behavior and *in vivo* tumorigenesis of the two NPC cell lines in athymic nude mice. Consistent with the hypothesis, we indeed observed that METCAM/MUC18 over-expression suppressed the tumor growth of NPC-TW01 cells, which were established from type I NPC [47], as previously shown [24, 25]. We thus conclude that METCAM/MUC18 plays a tumor suppressor role in the development of the type I NPC [24, 25].

Surprisingly, when a different cell line, NPC-TW04, was used for the similar set of the experiments we observed a completely opposite effect of METCAM/MUC18. We observed that over-expression of METCAM/MUC18 promoted *in vitro* and *in vivo* tumor growth of NPC-TW04 cells, which were established from type III NPC [47], as previously reported [24, 26]. We thus conclude that METCAM/MUC18 plays a tumor promoter role in the development of the type III NPC [24, 26].

Taken together we hypothesized that METCAM/MC18 plays a dual suppressor and promotor role in the different types of NPC.

3.3 Ovarian carcinoma

Two independent groups showed that METCAM/MUC18 expression is correlated with the progression of ovarian cancer [27, 48], and it affects the *in vitro* behaviors of ovarian carcinoma cells [49]. However, the role of METCAM/MUC18 in the progression of epithelial ovarian cancer has not been directly tested in animal models. To investigate this, we initiated the studies by testing the effect of over-expression of METCAM/MUC18 on the *in vitro* cellular behaviors and *in vivo* tumorigenesis and malignant progression of human ovarian cancer cell lines in nude mice. First, we used a human ovarian cell line, SK-OV-3, for testing the effects of METCAM/MUC18 expression on their *in vitro* motility and invasiveness, and *in vivo* tumor formation after subcutaneous (SC) injection and also *in vivo* progression after intraperitoneal (IP) injection in athymic nude mice. We observed that over-expression of METCAM/MUC18 reduced *in vitro* motility and invasiveness [28] and suppressed *in vivo* tumorigenesis and malignant progression of the human ovarian cancer cell line SK-OV-3 [28]. Then, we used the other human ovarian cancer cell line, BG-1, for similar tests and also observed similar phenomenon [50].

In summary, we supplied *in vitro* and *in vivo* evidence to definitely support the conclusion that METCAM/MUC18 plays a suppressor role in the tumorigenesis and malignant progression of two human ovarian cancer cell lines [28, 50]. Our results suggest that METCAM/MUC18 is a strong candidate as a new tumor and metastasis suppressor in human ovarian cancer cells.

3.4 Prostate cancer

For the previous two decades, we have firmly established the notion that over-expression of METCAM/MUC18 promotes the tumorigenesis and metastasis

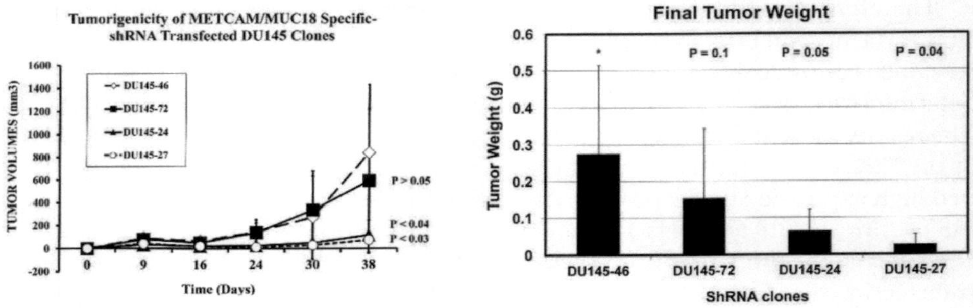

Figure 2.
Tumorigenicity of four shRNA-knockdown clones of DU145. Effect of METCAM/MUC18 expression on in vivo tumorigenicity (Left) and final tumor weight (Right). (Left) Average tumor volumes from five mice S.C. injected with each of the 46 (control), 72, 24, and 27 clones/cells, which were transfected with four corresponding shRNAs in pGIPZ vector, were plotted against time. (Right) Average final tumor weights from five mice S.C. injected with the same clones/cells and standard deviations were plotted at the end point of experiment. P values are shown in the figure by comparing the data to the control clone [51].

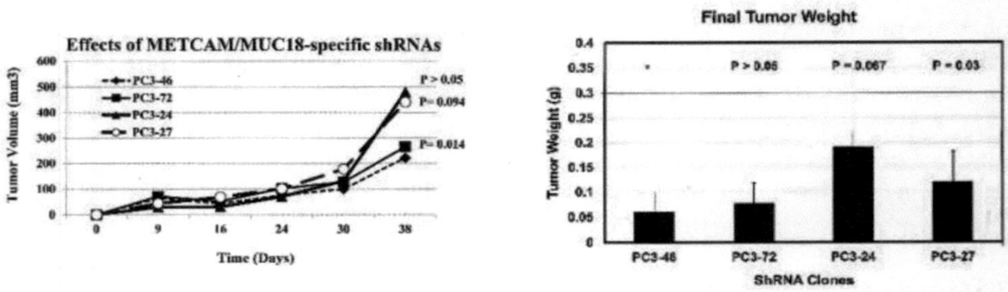

Figure 3.
Tumorigenicity of four shRNA-knockdown clones of PC-3. Effect of METCAM/MUC18 expression on in vivo tumorigenicity (Left) and final tumor weight (Right). (Left) Average tumor volumes from five mice S.C. injected with each of the 46 (control), 72, 24, and 27 clones/cells, which were transfected with the four corresponding shRNAs in pGIPZ vector, were plotted against time. (Right) Average final tumor weights from five mice S.C. injected with the same clones/cells and standard deviations were plotted at the end point of experiment. P values are shown in the figure by comparing the data to the control clone [52].

of human prostate cancer cell line LNCaP, which was established from lymphatic lesions [31–36]. To check if the conclusion is also extended to another human prostate cancer cell line DU145, we recently tested the effect of knocking down the endogenously expressed METCAM/MUC18 on tumorigenesis in a nude mouse system, since DU145 endogenously expressed a high level of METCAM/MUC18 [51]. We found that knocking down of the endogenously expressed METCAM/MUC18 with three shRNAs decreased the subcutaneous tumorigenesis in male nude mice in comparison to a control shRNA, as shown in **Figure 2**. We thus concluded that METCAM/MUC18 expression in DU145 cell line, which was established from brain lesions, plays a positive role in tumorigenesis (and perhaps metastasis) similar to in LNCaP cells.

In contrast, we recently used the similar knocking down strategy to test the effect of decreased the endogenous METCAM/MUC18 expression on *in vivo* tumorigenesis of another human prostate cancer cell line, PC-3, which was established from bone lesions, surprisingly we found that knocking down the endogenously expressed METCAM/MUC18 increased the tumor proliferation of PC-3 cells (which was opposite to that of DU145, as shown above in **Figure 2**), suggesting that expression of METCAM/MUC18 suppressed the tumorigenesis of the human prostate cancer cell line PC-3 [52], as shown in **Figure 3**.

Tumor/cancer cell lines	Tumorigenesis	Metastasis	References
Colorectal cancer human cell lines HT-29, SW480, SW948, SW620, colo205, Lovo320, P6C	Suppression	Not determined	[54]
Hemangioma human cell lines HemEC, HDMEC	Possible suppression	Not determined	[46]
Mouse melanoma cell line K1735-9	Suppression	Suppression	[22]
Mouse melanoma cell lines K1735-3, K1735-10	No effect or slight suppression	Increasing and affecting the late stage	[21]
Nasopharyngeal carcinoma type I cell line NPC-TW01	Suppression	Not determined	[24, 25]
Ovarian cancer cell lines SK-OV3, BG-1	Suppression	Suppression	[28, 50]
Pancreatic cancer human cell lines, UACC-1273, PANC1, C81-61, KP-2, SUIT-2, MIAPaca-2, HS766T and primary CAFs	Suppression	Suppression	[55, 56]
Prostate cancer human cell line PC-3	Suppression	Not determined	[52]

Table 1.
The negative role of METCAM/MUC18 in tumor formation and/or cancer metastasis of seven tumor/cancer cell lines.

We thus conclude that METCAM/MUC18 serves as a tumor suppressor in the PC-3 cell line, different from its role in two other prostate cancer cell lines (LNCaP and DU145), suggesting that prostate cancer cell lines established from different organs may have different intrinsic factors that modulate the function of METCAM/MUC18.

3.5 Colorectal cancer, hemangioma and pancreatic cancer

The protein METCAM/MUC18 is also expressed others cancers, such as angiosarcoma, gestational trophoblastic tumors, Kaposi's sarcoma, leiomyosarcoma, some lung squamous and small cell carcinomas, and some neuroblastoma [44]. However, its role in the development of most of these cancers is not well known. Recent meta-analysis suggests that high METCAM/MUC18 expression in many solid tumors appears to be associated with poor prognosis and patient survival [53]. However, in contrast to the conclusion, reduced expression of METCAM/MUC18 associates with the malignant progression of hemangioma [46]. Likewise, recent results of the effects of METCAM/MUC18 expression on tumorigenesis of colorectal cancer and pancreatic cancer also appear to support the similar conclusion, as described next. Reduced expression of METCAM/MUC18 promotes tumorigenesis and stemness of colorectal cancer [54]. Targeting soluble METCAM/MUC18 with a neutralizing antibody inhibits vascularization, growth and survival of METCAM/MUC18-positive pancreatic tumors [55]. Furthermore, attenuation of METCAM/MUC18 promotes pancreatic cancer progression [56]. Thus, the possible tumor and metastasis suppressor role of METCAM/MUC18 in solid tumors appear to extend from mouse melanoma K1735–9 subline, ovarian cancer, and NPC type I, to colorectal cancer [54] and pancreatic cancer [55, 56], and perhaps hemangioma [46]. **Table 1** summarizes the negative role of METCAM/MUC18 in the tumor formation and/or cancer metastasis of seven tumors/cancers.

4. METCAM/MUC18: a tumor promoter in most solid tumors

In contrast to the above functions of METCAM/MUC18, recent work done on other solid tumors appears to be consistent with the meta-analysis results of solid tumors [53],

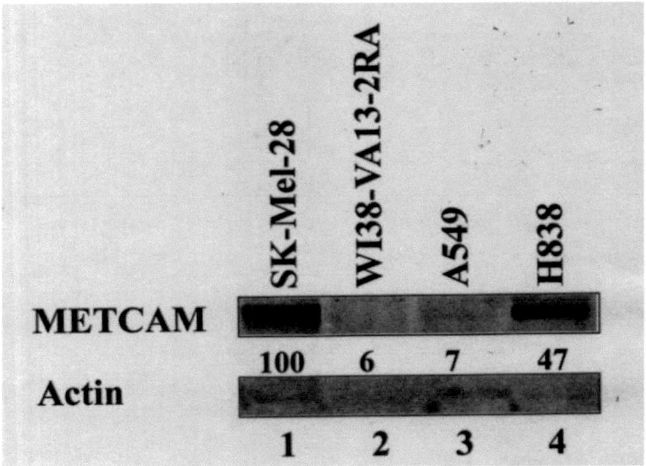

Figure 4.
Expression of METCAM/MUC18 in normal lung tissue (SV40-immortalized normal lung cells (WI38, lane 2) and lung type II alveolar epithelial cell carcinoma cell (A549, lane 3) and lung primary adenocarcinoma (H838, lane 4) (from Guang-Jer Wu, unpublished data).

as described next. For example, METCAM/MUC18 expression correlates with the epithelial-mesenchymal transition (EMT) markers and a poor prognosis in gastric cancer [57]. Tumor up-take of glioma in an orthotopic xenograft mouse model correlates with the expression level of METCAM/MUC18 [58]. METCAM/MUC18 promotes metastasis and predicts poor prognosis of hepatocellular carcinoma [59]. Increased expression of METCAM/MUC18 has been found in hepatocellular carcinoma (HCC) tumor tissues as compared with the matched adjacent normal liver tissues and the METCAM/MUC18$^+$ cells purified from HCC tumors and cells have significantly increased colony-forming capacity consistent with the cancer stem cells or the tumor-initiating cells [60]. METCAM/MUC18 expression has been shown to express in 51% of non-small cell lung carcinoma (NSCLC) and positive expression of METCAM/MUC18 has been associated with a shorter survival of patients with adenocarcinomas and used to predict the poor overall survival in patients with lung adenocarcinomas [61–63]. METCAM/MUC18 expression mediates acquisition of cancer stemness and enhances tumor invasion and metastasis in a mouse model [64]. High expression of METCAM/MUC18 correlates with intrapulmonary metastasis of NSCLC cells in a mouse model [65]. Consistent with the results, we showed in **Figure 4** (Guang-Jer Wu, unpublished data) that METCAM/MUC18 is expressed in a lung type II alveolar epithelial cell carcinoma cell, A549, and highly expressed in an adenocarcinoma cell line, H838, in comparison with its no expression in an immortalized normal embryonic WI38 cell line.

Furthermore, METCAM/MUC18 mediates chemoresistance of small cell lung carcinoma (SCLC) [66]. METCAM/MUC18 is expressed in osteosarcoma cell lines, but not in normal osteoblast cells [67]. Osteosarcoma is effectively treated with METCAM/MUC18 monoclonal antibodies [68, 69]. Transcription factor MEIS1 activates METCAM/MUC18 expression to promote migration of mouse pancreatic tumor cell lines [70]. METCAM/MUC18 very likely promotes the formation of angiosarcoma, as supported by our preliminary results as described next. Mouse METCAM/MUC18 was expressed in one angiosarcoma clone, SVR, which was transfected with H-Ras, at a higher level than in the control cell line, an immortalized normal endothelial cell line, MS-1 [71]. Furthermore, the tumorigenicity of the SVR cell line was higher than the control cell line, thus in direct association with the higher expression level of moMETCAM/MUC18 [40, 71]. This suggests that METCAM/MUC18 very likely promotes the formation of angiosarcoma [40, 71].

Tumor/cancer tissues or cell lines	Tumorigenesis	Metastasis	References
Angiosarcoma human cell lines MS1, SVR	Increasing	Not determined	[40, 71]
Human breast cancer cell line MCF-7	Promotion	Not determined	[18]
Human breast cancer cell line SK-BR-3	Promotion	Not determined	[19, 20]
Human breast cancer cell lines MDA-MB-231 and MDA-MB-468	Promotion	Promotion	[19, 45]
Gastric cancer human tissues	Promotion	Not determined	[57]
Glioma cell lines U87MG, U251	Promotion	Not Determined	[58]
Hepatocellular carcinoma human cell lines PLC/PRF/5, Huh7, MHCC97H& 97 L HepG2, SMMC-7721, focus, YY-8103, LM3, HLF and primary HCC cell lines; normal liver cell line LO2	Promotion	Not determined	[59, 60]
Non-small cell lung cancer human cell lines A549, H23, H358, H460, H522, H838, HCC4006, H1650/ER, PC-9, PC9GR, and adenocarcinoma tissues	Promotion	Promotion	[61–65], our unpublished results
Small cell lung cancer human cell lines H69, H69AR, H82, H196, H209, DMS79	Promotion	Not determined	[66]
Clinical melanoma tissues and human melanoma cell lines SB-2, SK, XP-44	No effect	Increasing and affecting the late stage	[38, 72, 73]
Mouse melanoma cell lines K1735-3, K1735-10	No effect or slight suppression	Increasing and affecting the late stage	[21]
Nasopharyngeal carcinoma type III human cell line NPC-TW04	Promotion	Not determined	[24, 26]
Osteosarcoma human cell lines CR9, MNNG-HOS, OHS, KPDX, KRIB, MG-63, shYY1, SaOS, SaOS-2, TE85, U20S	Promotion	Augmentation	[67–69]
Pancreatic cancer mouse cell lines ptf1a, LSL-Kras, LSL-Trp53, Pdx1,	Promotion	Possible augmentation	[70]
Clinical prostate cancer human tissues	Increasing	Increasing and affecting initiation in the early stage (PIN)	[31]
Human prostate cancer cell line LNCaP	Increasing	Increasing and affecting initiation in the early stage	[32, 34–36]
Human prostate cancer cell line DU145	Increasing	Not determined	[51]
Prostate adenocarcinoma in TRAMP mice	Increasing	Increasing and affecting initiation in the early stage	[33]

Table 2.
The positive role of METCAM/MUC18 in tumor formation and/or cancer metastasis of various tumors/cancers.

Hence, the positive role played by the METCAM/MUC18 in the progression of solid tumors have been extended from breast cancer, human and mouse melanoma, prostate cancer to angiosarcoma [40, 71], gastric cancer [57], glioma [58], hepatocellular carcinoma [59, 60], non-small cell lung adenocarcinoma [61–65], small cell lung cancer [66], osteosarcoma [67–69], and mouse pancreatic cancer [70]. Taken together, METCAM/MCU18 appears to be more prevalently in playing a positive role than a negative role in the tumorigenesis of solid tumors. **Table 2** summarizes the positive role of METCAM/MUC18 in the tumor formation and/or cancer metastasis of various tumors/cancers.

In conclusion, METCAM/MUC18 appears to play a dual role in the tumorigenesis and perhaps also in metastasis of solid tumors. At this point, it is not clear why METCAM/MUC18 plays a dual role in this aspect. Since METCAM/MUC18 only plays a dual role in different cell lines from the same type of cancer or in different type of cancers, but never in the same cancer cell line. It is logical to suggest a possible explanation that the intrinsic properties of each cancer cell line may provide specific co-factors or heterophilic ligands that may positively or negatively modulate the METCAM/MUC18-mediated tumorigenesis and metastasis. This can be readily scrutinized by identifying these specific intrinsic co-factors or heterophilic ligands by using immunological co-precipitation method in the future studies. This approach is feasible as described in one of the following sections, Section 5.1.

5. Putative mechanisms

Since the huMETCAM/MUC18 was first discovered in the 1980s, three groups have worked on the role of huMETCAM/MUC18 in melanoma metastasis [38, 39, 72, 73], another group on the role of huMETCAM/MUC18 in the biology of endothelial cells [41], and our group joined in the effort to study the role of huMETCAM/MUC18 in the progression of mouse melanoma [43] and prostate cancer [31–36, 51, 52], and later breast cancer [18–20], ovarian cancer [27–30], and NPC [23–26], as described above. Recently, more groups have participated in further exploring the possible role of METCAM/MUC18 in other solid tumors in different organs, such as colorectum [54], gastro-organ [57], glioma [58], liver [59, 60], lung [61–66], pancreas [55, 56, 70], and bone [67–69]. Preliminary work in leiomyosarcoma, esophagus squamous cell carcinoma, clear cell renal sarcoma, and gallbladder adenocarcinoma are also beginning to emerge [53].

After many decades of group effort, we are beginning to understand the biology of METCAM/MUC18-mediated tumor progression. However, the biological mechanisms describing the role of METCAM/MUC18 in tumorigenesis and malignant progression are still not well clarified such as: the protein's domain involved in cell adhesion, the domain which mediates the interactions of tumor cells with the tumor microenvironment leading to tumor progression and in the METCAM/MUC18-mediated tumorigenesis and malignant progression, and the effects of N-glycosylation on the functions of METCAM/MUC18 in tumorigenesis. Though the huMETCAM/MUC18-mediated outside-in and inside-out signaling in endothelial cells are understood to some extent, and the METCAM/MUC18-mediated signaling, which is leading to the progression of various cancer cells, are not much known. How METCAM/MUC18 is positively or negatively regulated at the level of transcription in different cancer cells remains minimally known. As such, the following five important aspects are much needed for immediate future studies, such as different kinds or quantities of co-factors or heterophilic ligand(s) in different cancer cell lines, contributions of different domains of the protein, different signaling pathways involved, differential regulation at the transcription level in tumors of different organs, and possible different extent of N-glycosylation in different cancer cell lines, which may critically modulate the function of METCAM/MUC18 in tumor progression.

5.1 The heterophilic ligands of METCAM/MUC18

The heterophilic ligands of METCAM/MUC18 may play an important role in the cell-cell and cell-extra-cellular matrix interactions and cancer metastasis. Our preliminary results suggest that the 72 kDa protein identified by immunoprecipitation method may be one of the heterophilic ligands for METCAM/MUC18, as shown in **Figure 5** [40].

As shown in **Figure 5**, the putative heterophilic ligand 72 kDa is highly expressed in the PC-3 cell line, but much less in the DU145 cell line. This may reveal a possible explanation for the different role of huMETCAM/MUC18 in the tumorigenicity of the two prostate cancer cell lines [40].

5.2 The domains of huMETCAM/MUC18 required for tumorigenesis and metastasis

The relation of the protein structure of huMETCAM/MUC18 to its functions in tumorigenesis and metastasis have not been systematically defined. To begin addressing this question, we have generated mutants deleted different domains of huMETCAM/MUC18 by using a special PCR method [74] and used them to determine their contribution to tumorigenesis. Surprisingly, our results showed that the ecto-domain of huMETCAM/MUC18 induced tumorigenesis in LNCaP cells in nude mice, as well as the whole wild type of cDNA. These preliminary results suggested

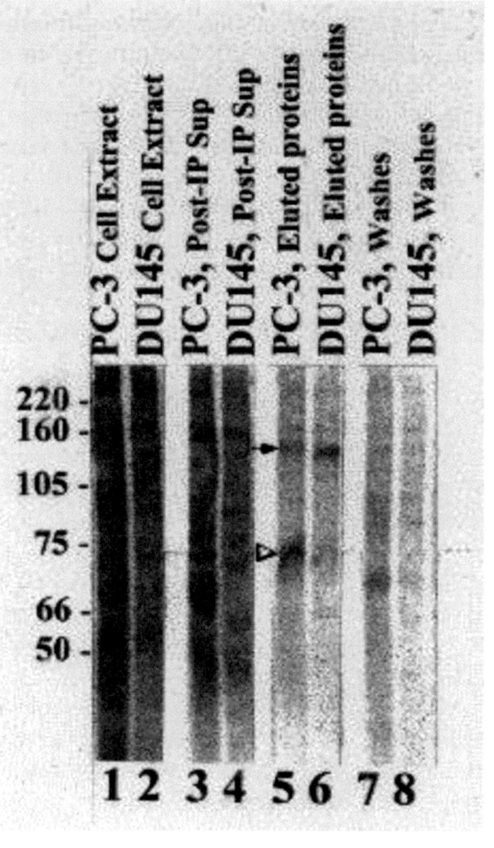

Figure 5.
Putative heterophilic ligand of METCAM/MUC18 in PC-3 and DU145 cell lines.

the key role of the ecto-domain in tumorigenesis induction in prostate cancer cells *in vivo*. This may implicate a puzzling notion that the cytoplasmic domain was not essential for this process (Guang-Jer Wu, data not shown). However, the critical direct test of using only the cytoplasmic domain for inducing tumor has not been performed for LNCaP cells. From the above puzzling observation, it is very clear that a systematic study has also to be performed in other cancer cell lines before a definitive conclusion can be drawn.

5.3 Signaling pathways in the METCAM/MUC18-mediated tumorigenesis and cancer metastasis

The huMETCAM/MUC18 contains three sites which are potentially phosphorylated by PKC, PKA and CK2 in the cytoplasmic tail [38, 42]. However, these putative phosphorylation sites have not been biochemically proven. Thus, the immediate question to be answered is that how many sites in the cytoplasmic tail of the native METCAM/MUC18 protein, which are to be isolated from different cancer cell lines, are actually phosphorylated? Which protein kinase is responsible for the phosphorylation? After this is answered, then we can further study how METCAM/MUC18 mediates crosstalk and networking with different signal pathways and to see if it is similar to or different from the cytoplasmic tails of other CAMs [41, 75–77]. Knowledge learned from other CAMs seem point to one aspect that METCAM/MUC18, as an integral membrane protein and a cell adhesion molecule, should mediate inside-in, inside-out, and outside-in signals to participate in intercellular communication and interaction of cell with extra-cellular matrix, which results in impacting cell motility and invasiveness [78, 79]. Furthermore, its interaction with co-factors or cognate heterophilic ligand(s) may alter these signals, which in turn should affect intrinsic tumor proliferation or impact tumor angiogenesis and/or mediate targeting to specific organs and promoting metastasis. Moreover, METCAM/MUC18 may interact with various hormonal receptors, growth or anti-growth factors/receptors, various chemokines/receptors, and the Ca^{2+}-mediated signaling members, which in turn affect the process of tumor progression. **Figure 6** summarizes the possible preliminary crosstalk of huMETCAM/MUC18 with many members of signal transduction pathways that may affect its function during tumor initiation and development and malignant progression.

5.4 Regulation of the huMETCAM/MUC18 gene transcription

The mechanism of transcriptional control of METCAM/MUC18 gene is minimally studied [17]. Up to now, only the 900 bp sequences in the core promoter region of the huMETCAM/MUC18 gene are well-characterized [80]. This core promoter is rich in GC sequences but does not contain a TATA box. It includes many consensus sequences presumably as putative binding sites for various transcription regulatory factors, such as SP-1, CREB [81], AP-2 [82, 83], c-Myb [84], N-Oct2 (Brn2) [85], Ets [86], CArG [87], and Egr-1 [88]. In addition, it also contains three insulin responsive elements (one Ets and two E-box motifs) [89], suggesting that huMETCAM/MUC18 gene expression may respond to the cue of various growth signals [37, 40], as shown in **Figure 7**.

In addition, some sequences upstream of the minimal core promoter sequences should also be expected for conferring the tissue-specific expression of the huMETCAM/MUC18 gene [90]. Recently this notion has been definitely supported by a finding that Ets sequence in the 10 kilo-bp up-stream region is involved in the regulation of the expression of huMETCAM/MUC18 gene [91]. We have also engaged in this task by searching the sequence of the up-stream region of the huMETCAM/MUC18 promoter in the Celera or other web sites. By taking advantage of the

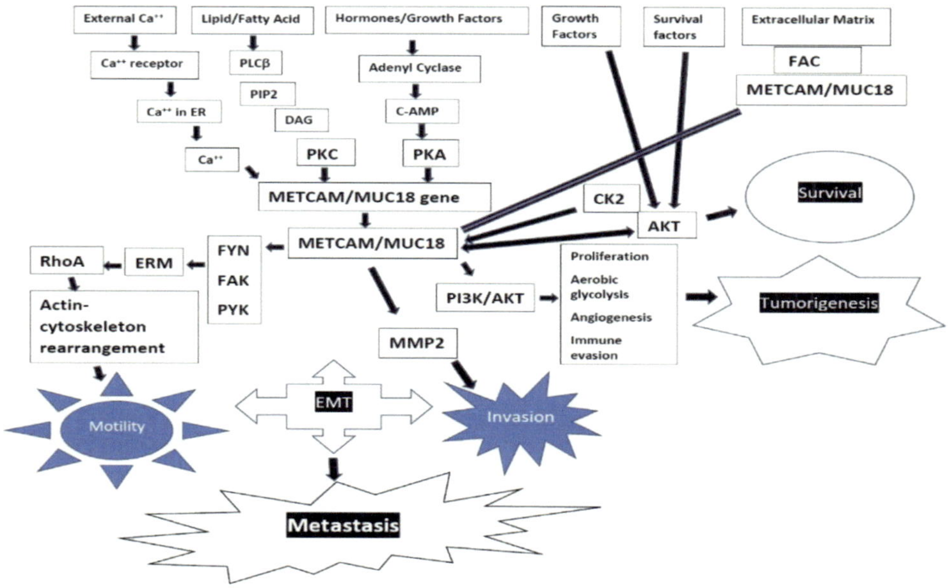

Figure 6.
METCAM/MUC18-mediated signal transduction in tumorigenesis and malignant progression.

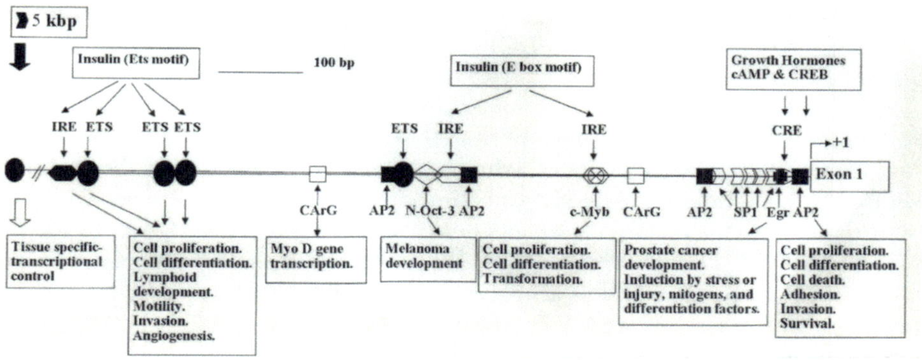

Figure 7.
Putative transcription factor-recognized motifs in the 900 bp core promoter and 5–10 kilo bp up-stream region of the huMETCAM/MUC18 gene.

known sequence searched, we designed many pairs of primers to screening a genomic library and obtained several phage clones which contain at least 4 kilo-bp of the gene for future studies (Guang-Jer Wu, unpublished data).

The epigenetic control of the expression of huMETCAM/MUC18 gene has not been extensively studied in NPC, though it has been implicated [92]. This is because huMETCAM/MUC18 gene is located at the locus of human chromosome 11q23.3 that has been shown to be hypermethylated in NPC, suggesting that the expression of this gene may be regulated by epigenetic controls [93]. To support this notion, our preliminary results of treating NPC cell lines with 5-Aza-2′-deoxycytidine (Aza-C) showed that after the treatment with Aza-C, METCAM/MUC18 expression was somewhat elevated in the NPC-TW01 cell line, but not in the NPC-TW04 cell line (Guang-Jer Wu, unpublished data). METCAM/MUC18 has also been shown to be methylated in most of the early stage of prostate cancer [94]. Further systematic studies in this aspect should be very interesting and rewarding in the future.

5.5 The possible roles of glycosylation on the protein of METCAM/MUC18 in tumorigenesis and tumor progression

Glycosylation of a protein may affect the proper folding, stability, and/or activity of a protein [95], however, the possible roles of glycosylation in the function of MCETCAM/MUC18 protein have not been explored. The glycosylation of METCAM/MUC18 may also affect its ability in inducing/promoting or suppressing the metastasis of cancer cells [95–99]. Both huMETCAM/MUC18 and moMETCAM/MUC18 may very likely to be heavily glycosylated, sialylated, and post-translationally modified, because both have an apparent molecular weight of about 110–150 kDa, which is much more than the naked protein with a molecular weight of about 65–70 kDa [100]. To initiate the study, we subjected the huMETCAM/MUC18, which was expressed in a human cancer cell line, to the digestion with N-glycosidase F, neuraminidase (sialidase), O-glycosidase, or endoglycosidase H, and we observed that the apparent molecular weight of the protein was decreased after digestion with N-glycosidase F and neuraminidase (sialidase), but not with O-glycosidase or endoglycosidase H [37, 40]. From this, we suggested that both sialic acid and N-glycans are probably the major carbohydrate side chains of huMETCAM/MUC18. It is also possible that glycosylation may differ depending on the type of cancers. Thus, we suggested that different N-glycans at the N-glycosylation sites of huMETCAM/MUC18 may differ in different cancer cell lines, which may have significant positive or negative impacts on their EMT abilities as well as tumorigenesis and metastasis. According to our hypothesis, a recent study described GCNT3 as an up-stream regulator of METCAM/MUC18. Moreover, GCNT3 glycosylates METCAM/MUC18 and extends its half-life which results in further elevation of S100A8/A9-mediated cellular motility in melanoma cells [101].

By searching in the primary sequence of the human huMETCAM/MUC18 protein, nine potential N-glycosylation sites (Asn-X-Ser/Thr or N-X-S/T sites) have been revealed [37, 38, 40, 42], whereas only seven sites found in the mouse METCAM/MUC18 [43]. Six N-glycosylation sites are conserved between the two proteins: 56/58 NL/FS, 418/420NRT, 449/451NLS, 467NGT/469NGS, 507NTS/509NTT, and 544/546NST [37, 38, 40, 42]. We suggest that only these six conserved N-glycosylation sites are actually glycosylated, because the apparent molecular weights of human METCAM/MUC18 and mouse METCAM/MUC18 are similar in the SDS gel. All the N-glycosylation sites are located in the external region of the protein, such as the domains of V1, C′, C″ and X. First, all these six sites should be biochemically identified before further molecular genetic task. Then, we will use genetic tools to alter the N-glycosylation sites. The mutants will be transfected back into cancer cell lines without the endogenous expression of the protein. The clones, which only express these mutated METCAM/MUC18, will be used for various *in vitro* and *in vivo* experiments to test the effect of N-glycosylation on the function huMETCAM/MUC18. They also will be used for testing effects on *in vitro* cell–cell aggregation and cell-extracellular matrix adhesion and on *in vivo* tumorigenesis and metastasis of human cancer cells. We anticipate that systematic studies on this aspect should be very informative to reveal the essential role of N-glycosylation played in the METCAM/MUC18-mediated tumor progression.

6. Conclusions

METCAM/MUC18 plays a key role in suppressing the progression of colorectal cancer, one mouse melanoma cell line, NPC type I, ovarian cancer, pancreatic cancer, prostate cancer PC-3 cell line, and perhaps hemangioma and possibly in other cancers.

On the other hand, METCAM/MUC18 also play a key positive function in the progression of breast cancer, gastric cancer, hepatocellular carcinoma, lung cancer, melanoma, NPC type III, pancreatic cancer, and prostate cancer. To further understand its role in these processes, it is essential to further identify its co-factor regulators and cognate heterophilic ligands, define its functional domains, and study its crosstalk with members of various signal transduction pathways, the regulation of its expression at the level of transcription, and effects of N-glycosylation on the functions of the protein.

7. Research perspectives and clinical applications

7.1 Research perspectives

The current studies have laid an important biological basis for inspiring future intense investigation to further understand the detailed knowledge of METCAM/MUC18-mediated suppression of tumorigenesis and metastasis of various cancer cell lines. For this purpose besides those have been described above, other future endeavors may include: (a) understanding three major mechanisms involved in METCAM/MUC18-induced tumor and metastasis dormancy, such as key players participated in inhibition of intrinsic growth capability, key chemokines and cytokines participated in suppression of immunological responses, and key pro-angiogenic and anti-angiogenic factors participated in the reduction of angiogenesis [102], (b) identification of possible miRNAs and non-coding RNAs participated in the process upstream and downstream of METCAM/MUC18 [103], and (c) possible clinical applications should be explored. Precaution should be taken that a complete picture may only be possibly constructed after all the above studies are successfully executed.

7.2 Clinical applications

The majority of the cancer-associated mortality is due to dissemination of primary tumor to distant organs (metastasis). If we are able to decrease or stop the metastatic propensity of cancer cells and keep them stayed only at the primary site, it should be a major success in cancer therapy. Alternatively, it is also a major success if we are able to control cancer cells at the state of dormancy or remaining them at the stage of micro-metastatic lesions [104]. Thus, similar to other tumor and metastasis suppressors, such as KISS1, KAI1, nm23, MAP2K4, and some micro-RNAs, METCAM/MUC18 may be used as a new therapeutic target for some clinical cancer treatments [105]. Strategically four major approaches may be taken for this purpose: (a) use gene therapeutic method to restore the functional copy of the suppressor genes or use epigenetic method to re-activate the genes. For gene therapy, the METCAM/MUC18 cDNA gene may be transported by an adenovirus-associated virus vector or a replication-defective adenovirus [106]. The human METCAM/MUC18 gene, located on 11q23-3 chromosome may be targeted with clinical reagents to reverse epigenetic repression, like Aza-C [107], or to change histone modifications to induce remodeling of the chromosome [108], (b) dispense recombinant proteins directly to the patients. For this approach, a complete copy or a partial portion of the METCAM/MUC18 recombinant protein, oligopeptides, or small molecule mimetics of METCAM/MUC18 may be directly dispensed to cancer patients, (c) target at downstream key members in the signaling pathways which are activated by the loss of the suppressor function, and (d) the co-factors or the cognate heterophilic ligand(s) of METCAM/MUC18 may be targeted. The above strategies may be used in single, or better in combination for treating the patients for the purpose of holding tumor cells at the primary sites, stopping them in a dormant state, or keeping the disseminating cancer cells at the state of micro-metastases. However, the dual role of METCAM/MUC18 in cancer progression may limit the above clinical applications to only cancers exhibiting an anti-tumor activity mediated by METCAM/MUC18.

Acknowledgements

I thank the support of grants from National Research Council, Taiwan.

Conflict of interests

The author has no conflict of interests.

Author details

Guang-Jer Wu

1 Department of Bioscience Technology, Center for Biomedical Technology, Chung Yuan Christian University, Taoyuan, Taiwan

2 Department of Microbiology and Immunology, Emory University School of Medicine, Atlanta, GA, USA

*Address all correspondence to: guangj.wu@gmail.com

References

[1] Jackson M, Marks L, May GHW, Wilson JB. The genetic basis of disease. Essays in Biochemistry. 2018;**62**:643-723

[2] Klinsmith LJ. Principles of Cancer Biology. San Francisco: Pearson Education Press; 2006

[3] Weinberg RA. The Biology of Cancer. 1st ed. New York, USA and Abington, UK: Garland Science; 2007

[4] Baylin SB, Jones PA. Epigenetic determinants in cancer. Cold Spring Harbor Perspectives in Biology. 2016;**8**(a019505):1-35

[5] Yang H, Villani RM, Wang H, Simpson MJ, Roberts MS, Tang M, et al. The role of cellular reactive oxygen species in chemotherapy. Journal of Experimental and Clinical Cancer Research. 2018;**37**(266):1-10

[6] Hanahan D, Weinberg RA. Hallmarks of cancer: The next generation. Cell. 2011;**144**:646-674. DOI: 10.1016/j.cell.2011.02.013

[7] Ramassone A, Pagotto S, Veronese A, Visone R. Epigenetics and MicroRNA in cancer. International Journal of Molecular Sciences. 2018;**19**(459):1-28

[8] Gkretsi V, Stylianopoulos T. Cell adhesion and matrix stiffness: Coordinating cancer cell invasion and metastasis. Frontiers in Oncology. 2018;**8**:145. DOI: 10.3389/fonc.2018.00145

[9] Mendonsa A, Na TY, Gumbiner BM. E-cadherin in contact inhibition and cancer. Oncogene. 2018;**37**(35):4769-4780

[10] Hamidi H, Ivaska J. Every step of the way: Integrins in cancer progression and metastasis. Nature Reviews. Cancer. 2018;**18**(9):533-548. DOI: 10.1038/s41568-018-0038-z

[11] Wang Z, Zhao K, Hackert T, Zoller M. CD44/CD44v6 a reliable companion in cancer-initiating cell maintenance and tumor progression. Frontiers in Cell and Development Biology. 2018;**6**:97. DOI: 10.3389/fcell.2018.00097

[12] Calinescu A, Turcu G, Nedelcu RI, Brinzea A, Hodorogea A, Antohe M, et al. On the dual role of carcinoembryonic antigen-related cell adhesion molecule 1 (CEACAM1) in human malignancies. Journal of Immunology Research. 2018;**2018**:ID7169081. 8p. DOI: 10.1155/2018/7169081

[13] Bhatia P, Gautqm SK, Cannon A, Thompson C, Hall BR, Aithal A, et al. Cancer-associated mucins: Role in immune modulation and metastasis. Cancer Metastasis Review. 9 Jan 2019. 14p. DOI:10.1007/s10555-018-09775-0

[14] Altevogt P, Doberstein K, Fogel M. L1CAM in human cancer. International Journal of Cancer. 2016;**138**:1565-1571

[15] Yahyazadeh Mashhadi SM, Kazemimanesh M, Arashkia A, Azadmanesh K, Meshkat Z, Golichenari B, et al. Shedding light on the EpCAM: An overview. Journal of Cellular Physiology. 2019;**234**(4):12569-12580

[16] Weidle UH, Eggle D, Klostermann S, Swart GWM. ALCAM/CD166: Cancer-related issues. Cancer Genomics and Proteomics. 2010;**7**(5):231-243

[17] Wu GJ. Chapter 13. Dual role of METCAM/MUC18 expression in the progression of cancer cells. In: Uchiumi F, editor. Gene Expression and Regulation in Mammalian Cells-Transcription from General Aspects. University Campus STeP Ri, Rijeka, Croatia: InTech Open Access Publisher; 2018. pp. 257-289.

ISBN 978-953-51-3856-3, Print ISBN 978-953-51-3855-6

[18] Zeng GF, Cai SX, Wu GJ. Up-regulation of METCAM/MUC18 promotes motility, invasion, and tumorigenesis of human breast cancer cells. BMC Cancer. 2011;**11**:113. DOI: 10.1186/1471-2407-11-113

[19] Zeng GF, Cai SX, Liu Y, Wu GJ. METCAM/MUC18 augments migration, invasion, and tumorigenicity of human breast cancer SK-BR-3 cells. Gene. 2012;**492**:229-238

[20] Huang CY, Wu GJ. METCAM/MUC18 promoted tumorigenesis of human breast cancer SK-BR-3 cells in a dosage-specific manner. Taiwanese Journal of Obstetrics and Gynecology. 2016;**55**(2):202-212. DOI: 10.1016/j.tjog.2016.02.010

[21] Wu GJ, Fu P, Wang SW, Wu MWH. Enforced expression of MCAM/MUC18 increases in vitro motility and invasiveness and in vivo metastasis of two mouse melanoma K1735 sublines in a syngeneic mouse model. Molecular Cancer Research. 2008;**6**(11):1666-1677

[22] Wu GJ. Ectopic expression of MCAM/MUC18 increases in vitro motility and invasiveness, but decreases in vivo tumorigenesis and metastasis of a mouse melanoma K1735-9 subline in a syngeneic mouse model. Clinical & Experimental Metastasis. 2016;**33**(8):817-828. DOI: 10.1007/s10585-016-9812-z

[23] Lin JC, Chiang CF, Wang SW, Wang WY, Kwuan PC, Wu GJ. Significance and expression of human METCAM/MUC18 in nasopharyngeal carcinoma (NPC) and metastatic lesions. Asian Pacific Journal of Cancer Prevention. 2014;**15**(1):245-252

[24] Liu YC. Putative roles of huMETCAM in modulating the development and progression of nasopharyngeal carcinoma [thesis]. Chung Yuan Christian University; 2014. Available from: http://www.lib.cycu.edu.tw/thesis

[25] Liu YC, Chen YR, Wu GJ. METCAM/MUC18 plays a tumor suppressor role in the development of nasopharyngeal carcinoma type I. 2019. (Submitted)

[26] Liu YC, Ke CC, Chen YR, Wu GJ. METCAM/MUC18 plays a tumor promoter role in the development of nasopharyngeal carcinoma type III. 2019. (Submitted)

[27] Wu GJ, Dickerson EB. Frequent and increased expression of human METCAM/MUC18 in cancer tissues and metastatic lesions associates with the clinical progression of human ovarian carcinoma. Taiwanese Journal of Obstetrics and Gynecology. 2014;**53**:509-517

[28] Wu GJ, Zeng GF. METCAM/MUC18 is a novel tumor and metastasis suppressor for the human ovarian cancer SKOV3 cells. BMC Cancer. 2016;**16**:136. DOI: 10.1186/S12885-016-2181-9

[29] Wu GJ. METCAM/MUC18 plays a novel tumor and metastasis suppressor role in the progression of human ovarian cancer cells. Obstetrics & Gynecology International Journal. 2017;**6**(4): 00210, pp. 1-8

[30] Wu GJ. METCAM/MUC18 decreases the malignant propensity of human ovarian carcinoma cells. International Journal of Molecular Sciences. 2018;**19**:02976

[31] Wu GJ, Varma VA, Wu MWH, Yang H, Wang SWC, Liu Z, et al. Expression of a human cell adhesion molecule, MUC18, in prostate cancer cell lines and tissues. The Prostate. 2001;**48**:305-315

[32] Wu GJ, Peng Q, Fu P, Chiang CF, Wang SWC, Dillehay DL, et al. Ectopical expression of human MUC18 increases metastasis of human prostate cancer LNCaP cells. Gene. 2004;**327**:201-213

[33] Wu GJ, Chiang CF, Fu P, Hess W, Greenberg N, Wu MWH. Increased expression of MUC18 correlates with the metastatic progression of mouse prostate adenocarcinoma in the (TRAMP) model. Journal of Urology. 2005;**173**:1778-1783

[34] Wu GJ, Wu MWH, Liu Y. Enforced expression of human METCAM/MUC18 increases the tumorigenesis of human prostate cancer cells in nude mice. Journal of Urology. 2011;**185**:1504-1512

[35] Wu GJ. Human METCAM/MUC18 as a novel biomarker to drive and its specific SiRNAs to block the malignant progression of prostate cancer. Journal of Cell Science and Therapy. 2015;**6**(5):1000227

[36] Wu GJ. Human METCAM/MUC18 is a new diagnostic marker of and a driver for promoting and its specific siRNAs, derived oligopeptides and antibodies be used for decreasing the malignant progression of prostate cancer. Journal of Stem Cell Research & Therapeutics. 2016;**1**(5):00035

[37] Wu GJ. Dual role of METCAM in the progression of different cancers. Journal of Oncology. 2012;**2012**:853797. DOI: 10.1155/2012/853797

[38] Lehmann JM, Reithmuller G, Johnson JP. MUC18, a marker of tumor progression in human melanoma. Proceedings of the National Academy of Sciences of the United States of America. 1989;**86**:9891-9895

[39] Meier F, Caroli U, Satyamoorthy K, Schittek B, Bauer J, Berking C, et al. Fibroblast growth factor-2 but not Mel-CAM and/or β3 integrin promotes progression of melanocytes to melanoma. Experimental Dermatology. 2003;**12**:296-306

[40] Wu GJ. METCAM/MUC18 expression and cancer metastasis. Current Genomics. 2005;**6**:333-349

[41] Anfosso F, Bardin N, Frances V, Vivier E, Camoin-Jau L, Sampol J, et al. Activation of human endothelial cells via S-Endo-1 antigen (CD146) stimulates the tyrosine phosphorylation of focal adhesion kinase p125FAK. The Journal of Biological Chemistry. 1998;**273**:26852-26858

[42] Wu GJ, Wu MWH, Wang SW, Liu Z, Peng Q, Qu P, et al. Isolation and characterization of the major form of human MUC18 cDNA gene and correlation of MUC18 over-expression in prostate cancer cells and tissues with malignant progression. Gene. 2001;**279**:17-31

[43] Yang H, Wang SWC, Liu Z, Wu MWH, McAlpine B, Ansel J, et al. Isolation and characterization of murine MUC18 cDNA gene, and correlation of MUC18 expression in murine melanoma cell lines with metastatic ability. Gene. 2001;**265**:133-145

[44] Shih IM. The role of CD146 (Mel-CAM) in biology and pathology. Journal of Pathology. 1999;**189**:4-11

[45] Zeng Q, Li W, Lu D, Wu Z, Duan H, Luo Y, et al. CD146, an epithelial-mesenchymal transition inducer, is associated with triple-negative breast cancer. Proceedings of the National Academy of Sciences of the United States of America. 2012;**109**(4):1127-1132

[46] Li Q, Yu Y, Bischoff J, Milliken JB, Olsen BR. Differential expression of CD146 in tissues and endothelial cells derived from infantile hemangioma and normal human skin. Journal of Pathology. 2003;**201**:296-302

[47] Lin CT, Wong CI, Chan WY, et al. Establishment and characterization of two nasopharyngeal carcinoma cell lines. Laboratory Investigation. 1990;**62**:713-724

[48] Aldovini D, Demichelis F, Doglioni C, Di Vizio D, Galligioni E, et al. M-CAM expression as marker of poor prognosis in epithelial ovarian cancer. International Journal of Cancer. 2006;**119**(8):1920-1926

[49] Wu Z, Wu ZY, Li J, Yang X, Wang Y, et al. MCAM is a novel metastasis marker and regulates spreading, apoptosis and invasion of ovarian cancer cells. Tumor Biology. 2012;**33**:1619-1628

[50] Wu GJ. Enforced expression of METCAM/MUC18 decreases in vitro motility and invasiveness and tumorigenesis and in vivo tumorigenesis of human ovarian cancer BG-1 cells. In: Schatten H, editor. Ovarian Cancer: Molecular & Diagnostic Imaging and Treatment Strategies, Advances in Experimental Medicine and Biology. Humana Press (Springer Science + Business Media LLC); 2019. (In press)

[51] Wu G-J, Chang YR, Chu JT. METCAM/MUC18 plays a positive role in the tumorigenesis of human prostate cancer DU145 cells: Knockdown effects shRNAs decreasing tumorigenicity in nude mice. 2019. (Submitted)

[52] Wu G-J, Chang YR, Chu JT. METCAM/MUC18 plays a negative role in the tumorigenesis of human prostate cancer PC-3 cells: Knockdown effects shRNAs increasing tumorigenicity in nude mice. 2019. (Submitted)

[53] Zeng P, Li H, Lu PH, Zhou LN, Tang M, Liu CY, et al. Prognostic value of CD146 in solid tumor: A systematic review and meta-analysis. Scientific Reports. 2017;**7**(1):4223. DOI: 10.1038/s41598-017-01061-3

[54] Liu D, Du L, Chen D, Ye Z, Duan H, Tu T, et al. Reduced CD146 expression promotes tumorigenesis and cancer stemness in colorectal cancer through activating Wnt/β-catenin signaling. Oncotarget. 2016;7(26):40704-40718

[55] Stalin J, Nollet M, Garigue P, Fernandez S, Vivavancos L, Essaah A, et al. Targeting soluble CD146 with a neutralizing antibody inhibits vascularization, growth, and survival of CD146 positive tumors. Oncogene. 2016;**35**:5489-5500

[56] Zheng B, Ohuchida K, Chijiiwa Y, Zhao M, Mizuuchi Y, Cui L, et al. CD146 attenuation in cancer-associated fibroblasts promotes pancreatic cancer progression. Molecular Carcinogenesis. 2016;**55**(11):1560-1572

[57] Liu WF, Ji SR, Sun JJ, Zhang Y, Liu ZY, Liang AB, et al. Gastric cancer CD146 expression correlates with epithelial-mesenchymal transition markers and a poor prognosis in gastric cancer. International Journal of Molecular Sciences. 2012;**13**:6399-6406

[58] Yang Y, Hernandez R, Rao J, Yin L, Qu Y, Wu J, et al. Targeting CD146 with a ^{64}Cu-labeled antibody enables in vivo immunoPET imaging of high-grade gliomas. Proceedings of the National Academy of Sciences of the United States of America. 2015;**112**(47):E6525-E6534

[59] Jiang G, Zhang L, Zhu Q, Bai D, Zhang C, Wang X. CD146 promotes metastasis and predicts poor prognosis of hepatocellular carcinoma. Journal of Experimental & Clinical Cancer Research. 2016;**35**:38. DOI: 10.1186/s13046-016-0313-3

[60] Chen K, Ding A, Ding Y, Ghanekar A. High-throughput flow cytometry screening of human hepatocellular carcinoma reveals CD146 to be a novel marker of tumor-initiating cells. Biochemistry and Biophysics Reports. 2016;**8**:107-113

[61] Kristiansen G, Yu Y, Schlüns K, Sers C, Dietel M, Petersen I. Expression of the cell adhesion molecule CD146/MCAM in non-small cell lung cancer. Analytical Cellular Pathology. 2003;**25**:77-81

[62] Oka S, Uramoto H, Chikaishi Y, Tanaka F. The expression of CD146 predicts a poor overall survival in patients with adenocarcinoma of the lung. Anticancer Research. 2012;**32**:861-864

[63] Zhang X, Wang Z, Kang Y, Li X, Ma X, Ma L. MCAM expression is associated with poor prognosis in non-small cell lung cancer. Clinical and Translational Oncology. 2014;**16**:178-183

[64] Zhang F, Wang J, Wang X, Wei N, Liu H, Zhang X. CD146-mediated acquisition of stemness phenotype enhances tumor invasion and metastasis after EGFR-TKI resistance in lung cancer. Clinical Respiratory Journal. 2019;**13**(1):23-33

[65] England CG, Jiang D, Hernandez R, Sun H, Valdovinos HF, Ehlerding EB, et al. ImmunoPET imaging of CD146 in murine models of intrapulmonary metastasis of non-small cell lung cancer. Molecular Pharmaceutics. 2017;**14**(10):3239-3247

[66] Tripathi SC, Fahrmann JF, Celiktas M, Aguilar M, Marini KD, Jolly MK, et al. A novel mechanism of chemoresistance in small cell lung cancer mediated by MCAM via PI3K/AKT/SOX2 signaling pathway. Cancer Research. 2017;**77**(16):4414-44252

[67] Schiano C, Grimaldi V, Casamassimi A, Infante T, Esposito A, Giovane A, et al. Different expression of CD146 in human normal and osteosarcoma cell lines. Medical Oncology. 2012;**29**(4):2998-3002

[68] McGary EC, Heimberger A, Mills L, Weber K, Thomas GW, Shtivelband M, et al. A fully human anti-melanoma cellular adhesion molecule/MUC18 antibody inhibits spontaneous pulmonary metastasis of osteosarcoma cells in vivo. Clinical Cancer Research. 2003;**9**:6560-6566

[69] Westrøm S, Bønsdorff TB, Abbas N, Bruland ØS, Jonasdottir TJ, Mælandsmo GM, et al. Evaluation of CD146 as target for radioimmunotherapy against osteosarcoma. PLoS One. 2016;**11**(10):e0165382. DOI: 10.1371/journal.pone.0165382

[70] von Burstin J, Bachhuber F, Paul M, Schmid RM, Rustgi AK. The TALE homeodomain transcription factor MEIS1 activates the pro-metastatic melanoma cell adhesion molecule MCAM to promote migration of pancreatic cancer cells. Molecular Carcinogenesis. 2017;**56**(3):936-944

[71] LaMontagne KR Jr, Moses MA, Wiederschain D, Mahajan S, Holden J, Ghazizadeh H, et al. Inhibition of MAP kinase causes morphological reversion and dissociation between soft agar growth and in vivo tumorigenesis in angiosarcoma cells. American Journal of Pathology. 2000;**157**:1937-1945

[72] Xie S, Luca M, Huang S, Gutman M, Reich R, Johnson JP, et al. Expression of MCAM/MCU18 by human melanoma cells leads to increased tumor growth and metastasis. Cancer Research. 1997;**57**:2295-2303

[73] Schlagbauer-Wadl H, Jansen B, Muller M, Polterauer P, Wolff K, Eichler HG, et al. Influence of MUC18/MCAM/CD146 expression on human melanoma growth and metastasis in SCID mice. International Journal of Cancer. 1999;**81**:951-955

[74] Geiser M, Cebe R, Drewello D, Schmitz R. Integration of PCR fragments at any specific site within cloning vectors without the use of

restriction enzymes and DNA ligase. BioTechniques. 2001;**31**:88-92

[75] Morgan MR, Thomas GJ, Russell A, Hart IR, Marshall JF. The integrin cytoplasmic tail motif EKQKVDLSTDC is sufficient to promote tumor cell invasion mediated by matrix metalloproteinase MMP-2 or MMP-9. The Journal of Biological Chemistry. 2004;**279**:26533-26539

[76] Heiz M, Grunberg J, Schubiger PA, Novak-Hofer I. Hepatocyte growth factor-induced ectodomain shedding of cell adhesion molecule L1-role of the cytoplasmic domain. The Journal of Biological Chemistry. 2004;**279**:31149-31156

[77] Anfosso F, Bardin N, Vivier E, Sabatier F, Sampol J, Dignat-George F. Outside-in signaling pathway linked to CD146 engagement in human endothelial cells. The Journal of Biological Chemistry. 2001;**276**:1564-1569

[78] Sastry SK, Horwitz AF. Integrin cytoplasmic domains: Mediators of cytoskeletal linkages and extra- and intracellular initiated transmembrane signaling. Current Opinion in Cell Biology. 1993;**5**:819-831

[79] Schoenwaelder SM, Burridge K. Bidirectional signaling between the cytoskeleton and integrins. Current Opinion in Cell Biology. 1999;**11**:274-286

[80] Sers C, Kirsch K, Rothbacher U, Riethmuller G, Johnson JP. Genomic organization of the melanoma-associated glycoprotein MUC18: Implications for the evolution of the immunoglobulin domains. Proceedings of the National Academy of Sciences of the United States of America. 1993;**90**:8514-8518

[81] Rummel MM, Sers C, Johnson JP. Phorbol ester and cyclic AMP-mediated regulation of the melanoma-associated cell adhesion molecule MUC18/MCAM. Cancer Research. 1996;**56**:2218-2223

[82] Jean D, Gershenwald JE, Huang S, Luca M, Hudson MJ, Tainsky MA, et al. Loss of AP-2 results in up-regulation of CAM/MUC18 and an increase in tumor growth and metastasis of human melanoma cells. The Journal of Biological Chemistry. 1998;**273**:16501-16508

[83] Ruiz M, Pettaway C, Song R, Stoeltzing O, Ellis L, Bar-Eli M. Activator protein 2a inhibits tumorigenicity and represses vascular endothelial growth factor transcription in prostate cancer cells. Cancer Research. 2004;**64**:631-638

[84] Ness SA. The Myb oncoprotein: Regulating a regulator. Biochimica et Biophysica Acta. 1996;**1299**:F123-F139

[85] Thomson JAF, Murphy K, Baker E, Sutherland GR, Parsons PG, Sturm RA. The brn-2 gene regulates the melanocytic phenotype and tumorigenic potential of human melanoma cells. Oncogene. 1995;**11**:691-700

[86] Yordy JS, Li R, Sementchenko VI, Pei H, Muise-Helmericks RC, Watson DK. S100 expression modulates ETS1 transcriptional activity and inhibits cell invasion. Oncogene. 2004;**23**:6654-6665

[87] L'honore A, Lamb NJ, Vandromme M, Turowski P, Carnac G, Fernandez A. MyoD distal regulatory region contains an SF binding CArG element required for MyoD expression in skeletal myoblasts and during muscle regeneration. Molecular Biology of the Cell. 2003;**14**:2151-2162

[88] Baron V, Duss S, Rhim J, Mercola D. Antisense to the early growth response-1 gene (Egr-1) inhibits prostate tumor development in TRAMP mice. Annals of the New York Academy of Sciences. 2003;**1002**:197-216

[89] O'Brien RM, Streeper RS, Ayala JE, Stadelmaier BT, Hornbuckle LA. Insulin-regulated gene expression. Biochemical Society Transactions. 2001;**29**:552-558

[90] Johnson JP, Rummel MM, Rothbacher U, Sers C. MUC18: A cell adhesion molecule with a potential role in tumor growth and tumor cell dissemination. Current Topics in Microbiology and Immunology. 1997;**213**:95-106

[91] Sechler M, Parrish JK, Birks DK, Jedlicka P. The histone demethylase KDM3A, and its downstream target MCAM, promote Ewing Sarcoma cell migration and metastasis. Oncogene. 2017;**36**(29):4150-4160

[92] Lung HL, Cheng Y, Kumaran MK, et al. Fine mapping of the 11Q22-23 tumor suppressive region and involvement of TSLC1 in nasopharyngeal carcinoma. International Journal of Cancer. 2004;**112**:628-635

[93] Wu GJ. MCAM (melanoma cell adhesion molecule). Atlas of Genetics and Cytogenetics in Oncology and Haematology (Open Access Journal). 2012. DOI: 10.4267/2042/47418. ID41314ch11q23. The manually annotated Biomax Human Genome Database Version 4.0, Biomax Informatics AG, www.biomax.com, the Biomax Solutions Inc., Falmouth, MA, USA

[94] Brait M, Banerjee M, Maldonado L, Ooki A, Loyo M, Guida E, et al. Promoter methylation of MCAM, ERα and ERβ in serum of early stage prostate cancer patients. Oncotarget. 2017;**8**(9):15431-15440. DOI: 10.18632/oncotarget.14873

[95] Parodi A. Protein glycosylation and its role in protein folding. Annual Review of Biochemistry. 2000;**69**:69-93

[96] Varki A. Glycosylation changes in tumor cells. In: Varki A, Cumming R, Esko J, Freeze H, Hart G, Marth J, editors. Essentials of glycobiology. NY: Cold Spring Harbor Laboratory Press; 1999. pp. 537-549

[97] Fukuda M. Possible roles of tumor-associated carbohydrate antigens. Cancer Research. 1996;**56**:2237-2244

[98] Hakomori S. Tumor malignancy defined by aberrant glycosylation and sphingo(glyco) lipid metabolism. Cancer Research. 1996;**56**:5309-5318

[99] Yamamoto H, Oviedo A, Sweeley C, Saito T, Moskal JR. α2,6-sialylation of cell-surface N-glycans inhibits glioma formation in vivo. Cancer Research. 2001;**61**:6822-6829

[100] Lehmann JM, Holzmann B, Breitbart EW, Schmiegelow P, Riethmuller G, Johnson JP. Discrimination between benign and malignant cells of melanocytic lineage by two novel antigens, a glycoprotein with a molecular weight of 113,000 and a protein with a molecular weight of 76,000. Cancer Research. 1987;**47**:841-845

[101] Sumardika W, Youyi C, Kondo E, Inoue Y, Ruma MW, Murata H, et al. β-1,3-galactosyl-O-glycosyl-glycoprotein β-1,6-N-acetylglucosaminyltransferase 3 increases MCAM stability, which enhances S100A8/A9-mediated cancer motility. Oncology Research. 2018;**26**(3):431-444

[102] Aguirre-Chiso JA. Models, mechanisms and clinical evidence for cancer dormancy. Nature Reviews. Cancer. 2007;**7**:834-846

[103] Kasinski AL, Slack FJ. MicroRNAs en route to the clinic: Progress in validating and targeting microRNAs for cancer therapy. Nature Reviews. Cancer. 2011;**11**:849-864

[104] Wikman H, Vessella R, Pantel K. Cancer micro-metastasis and tumor dormancy. APMIS. 2008;**116**:754-770

[105] Smith SC, Theodorescu D. Learning therapeutic lessons from metastasis suppressor proteins. Nature Reviews. Cancer. 2009;**9**(4):253-264

[106] Naldini L. Gene therapy returns to center stage. Nature. 2015;**526**(7573):351-360. DOI: 10.1038/nature15818

[107] Liang G, Weisenberger DJ. DNA methylation aberrancies as a guide for surveillance and treatment of human cancers. Epigenetics. 2017;**12**(6):416-432

[108] Shanmugam MK, Arfuso F, Arumugam S, Chinnathambi A, Jinsong B, Warrier S, et al. Role of novel histone modifications in cancer. Oncotarget. 2018;**9**(11):11414-11426

Section 2

Genes with Dual Tumor Suppressor and Oncogenic Activities

Chapter 3

Tumour Suppressor Genes with Oncogenic Roles in Lung Cancer

Mateus Camargo Barros-Filho, Florian Guisier,
Leigha D. Rock, Daiana D. Becker-Santos, Adam P. Sage,
Erin A. Marshall and Wan L. Lam

Abstract

Lung cancer is one of the most common cancers and the leading cause of cancer-related deaths worldwide. High-throughput sequencing efforts have uncovered the molecular heterogeneity of this disease, unveiling several genetic and epigenetic disruptions driving its development. Unlike oncogenes, tumour suppressor genes negatively regulate cell cycle control and exhibit loss-of-function alterations in cancer. Although tumour suppressor genes are more frequently disrupted, oncogenes are more likely to be drug-targeted. Many genes are described as presenting both tumour suppressive and oncogenic functions in different tumour types or even within the natural history of the disease in a single tumour. In this chapter, we describe current knowledge of tumour suppressor genes in lung tissues, focusing on tumour suppressor/oncogene duality.

Keywords: tumour-suppressor genes, oncogenes, dual roles, lung cancer, targeted therapy

1. Introduction

Cancer cells arise in non-malignant tissue due to the sequential acquisition of molecular alterations that drive proliferation, permit the evasion of growth suppression and apoptosis signals and promote angiogenesis, invasion and metastasis [1]. This process is stochastic, and over time the tumour continues to evolve in a dynamic manner, generating a group of cells harbouring different genetic and epigenetic features [2]. The resulting heterogeneity is the basis of tumour evolution and leads to the selection of tumour cells. These cells often present with rewired signalling networks and often oncogene addiction [3].

The uncontrolled growth of cancer cells can in part be explained by their aberrant gene expression patterns. While most cancer genes are characterized as either oncogenes or tumour suppressors based on their typical behaviour in tumours, some genes display dual oncogenic and tumour suppressive functions [4, 5]. The majority of these genes encode multiple isoforms, which are further post-translationally modified and form a variety of protein complexes, generating a context-dependent cellular network [6]. In diploid organisms, gain-of-function (GOF) mutations in oncogenes are typically dominant (single events are sufficient to promote tumourigenesis), while loss-of-function alterations are recessive in TSGs (requires two inactivation events) [7]. For example, for a TSG with dual oncogenic roles, one gain-of-function mutation can potentially cease its tumour suppressive function and turn on oncogenic signalling [5].

Recently, genes with both oncogenic and tumour-suppressive functions were described across 12 main cancer types using The Cancer Genome Atlas (TCGA) database [5]. Using a text mining approach, the authors identified genes mainly represented by kinases (e.g. *BCR*, *CHEK2*, *MAP2K4*, *NTRK3* and *SYK*) or transcription factors (e.g. *BRCA1*, *EZH2*, *NOTCH1*, *NOTCH2*, *STAT3* and *TP53*) and evaluated them at the genomic and gene expression levels. Using an *in silico* analysis, it was shown that genes with dual functions interact with more partners and are more important hub-genes in protein-protein interaction networks.

In this chapter, we discuss TSGs with both tumour suppressive and oncogenic functions in lung cancer.

1.1 Lung cancer classification

Lung cancer is one of the most common cancers and the leading cause of cancer-related deaths worldwide [8]. In the United States, lung cancer accounts for 13.5% of all new cancer cases and 25.3% of all cancer deaths. The five-year survival rate is dismal, with only 18.6% of patients surviving 5 years [9]. The majority of lung cancer cases (approximately 80%) are attributed to cigarette smoking [10]. About 10–25% of cases occur in people who have never smoked [11]. The aetiology behind these cases is most likely a combination of genetic factors, as well as the effects of exposure to environmental carcinogens such as asbestos, radon gas or other forms of pollution [12].

Lung cancer is classified according to histological type. There are two major types: small cell lung cancer (SCLC), which accounts for 15–20% of lung cancer patients, and non-small cell lung cancer (NSCLC), comprising the remaining 80–85% (**Figure 1**) [13]. SCLC, primarily originating from the central airways, is thought to be derived from neuroendocrine cells [14]. NSCLC is composed of three major histological

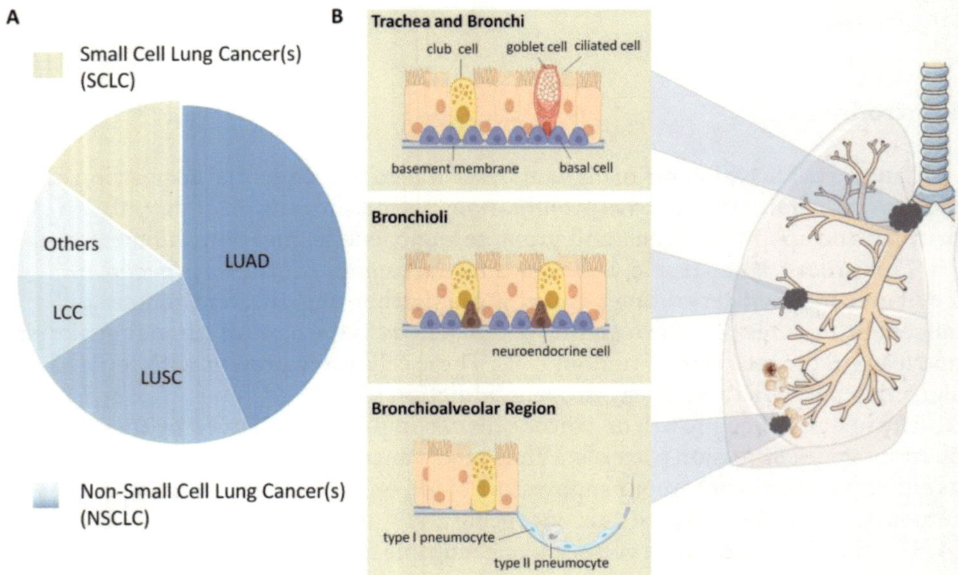

Figure 1.
Histological classification of lung cancer. (A) Lung cancer histological types. (B) Location of the tumours and cell origins. SCLC, small cell lung cancer; NSCLC, non-small cell lung cancer; LUAD, lung adenocarcinoma; LUSC, lung squamous cell carcinoma; LCC, large cell carcinoma.

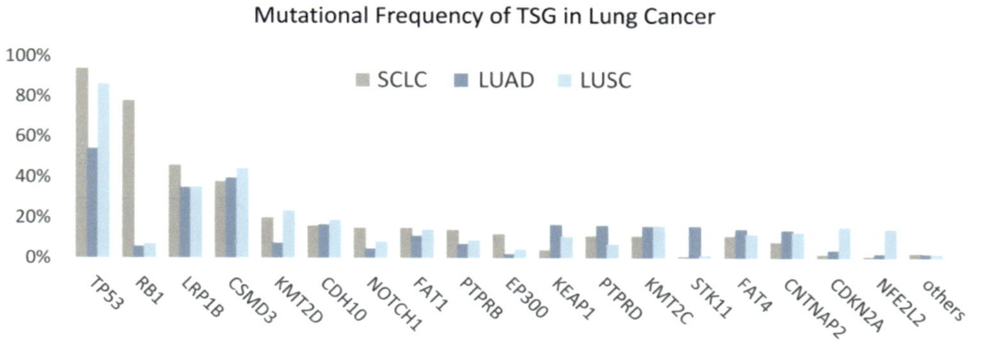

Figure 2.
Mutational frequency of TSGs in small cell lung cancer (SCLC; n = 110) [16], lung adenocarcinoma (LUAD; n = 660) [23] and lung squamous cell carcinoma (LUSC; n = 484) [23]. TSGs were defined according to COSMIC Cancer Gene Census (https://cancer.sanger.ac.uk/census) and mutation frequency of the most commonly disrupted TSGs in these subtypes of lung cancer were retrieved using cBioPortal (http://www.cbioportal.org/).

subtypes: adenocarcinoma (LUAD), squamous cell carcinoma (LUSC) and large cell carcinoma (LCC). LUAD is the most common, accounting for approximately 40% of all lung cases [15]. LUAD typically arises from glandular epithelium, from bronchioalveolar stem cells, club (Clara) cells or type II pneumocytes in the lung periphery [13]. LUAD is also the predominant subtype that arises in patients who have never smoked [15]. LUSC develops primarily in the central airways and segmental bronchi, strongly associates with a history of smoking and accounts for approximately 20% of all lung cancer cases. LCC may arise anywhere in the lung and are classified as tumours without general features associated with SCLC, LUAD or LUSC [13].

1.2 TSG mutation spectrum in lung cancer

Beyond the histological heterogeneity of lung cancer, genomic studies of large cohorts have uncovered the complex molecular landscape of lung tumours. Indeed, it has been observed that a wide variety of oncogenes and TSGs can be altered in lung cancer, and these molecular events are vastly different between histological subtypes [16, 17].

Clinical studies have shown that molecularly defined lung cancer subgroups can correlate with characteristics such as ethnicity [18], smoking history [19], treatment sensitivity [20] or prognosis [21]. Many of the commonly identified gain-of-function alterations in proto-oncogenes have been actively investigated for therapeutic purposes. For example, *EGFR, ALK, ROS1, BRAF, MET, RET* and *HER2* are routinely assessed in the clinic to offer targeted therapy for eligible LUAD patients [22].

Three TSGs are frequently mutated in all three major lung cancer subtypes: *TP53, LRP1B* and *CSMD3*. Other TSGs of particular interest in lung cancer are as follows *RB1* and *CREBBP* in SCLC, *KEAP1* and *STK11* in LUAD, *CDKN2A* in LUSC, *NOTCH1* and *PTEN* in both SCLC and LUSC and NF1 in both LUAD and LUSC (**Figure 2**). Mutations in these TSGs are usually mutually exclusive, indicating that individual genes are capable of driving lung cancer progression.

2. TSGs with oncogenic roles in lung cancer

Several TSGs in lung cancer have also been shown to behave as oncogenes, depending on the molecular context and/or the mechanism by which they are altered (**Table 1**). Among them are *TP53*, *NFIB*, members of the NOTCH family, *NKX2-1*, *NFE2L2*, as well as some non-coding RNAs (*MALAT1*, *mir*-125, and *mir*-378), which will be discussed in detail below.

2.1 *TP53*

TP53 is a well-known TSG, representing the most common somatically mutated gene in human cancer, especially in lung tumours [24]. The classic functions of the encoded p53 protein are cell cycle regulation, DNA repair, senescence mediated by stress, apoptosis and angiogenesis. These functions mainly occur through

Gene	Main function	Role as TSG	Role as oncogene
TP53	TF: regulates cell cycle, DNA repair, senescence and apoptosis	TSG in several tissues: frequently lost through mutations [24]	Missense mutations confer gain-of-function oncogenic properties [31]
NFIB	TF: crucial in lung development	Underexpressed in NSCLC and associated with poor survival in LUAD [32]	Amplified and OE in SCLC: inducing chromatin reprogramming during metastasis [33]
NOTCH1/NOTCH2	Transmembrane receptors: proliferation, differentiation and survival	Inactivated by inhibitor ligands and through mutations, especially in SCLC [34]	Maintains stem cell features; promotes proliferation in LUAD [35]
NFE2L2	TF: cellular defense mechanism against oxidative stress	Protects lung tissue against exposure to oxidative stress [36]	Mutational activation: aids cells to escape from endogenous tumour suppression [37]
NKX2-1	TF: essential for lung development	Acts as a TSG in *KRAS*-driven p53-mutant LUAD [38]	Enhanced oncogenic signals in *EGFR*-driven LUAD [39]
STK11	Serine-threonine kinase: regulation of energetic metabolism and cell polarity	Mutational inactivation promotes cancer development [40]	OE maintains metabolic homeostasis and attenuates oxidative stress [40]
TGFB	Cytokine: regulates development, differentiation and homeostasis	Expression loss leads to growth arrest in early-stage lung and other cancers [41]	OE promotes tumour growth in advanced cancer stages [42]
TUSC3	Endoplasmic reticulum protein in magnesium uptake, glycosylation and embryonic development	Hypermethylation; expression loss in NSCLC; inhibits cell proliferation and promotes apoptosis [43]	OE in NSCLC accelerates cancer growth; induces EMT [44]
WT1	TF: role in urogenital system development	Loss of function enhances cell viability and proliferation in Wilms' tumour [45]	OE promotes survival in *KRAS*-mutated NSCLC [46]
MALAT1	Long non-coding RNA	OE reduces invasiveness in PTEN expressing tumours [47]	OE associated with chemotherapy resistance in NSCLC [48]
miR-125b	microRNA	OE induces apoptosis [49]	OE promotes metastasis [50]
miR-378	microRNA	OE reverses chemoresistance to cisplatin in LUAD [51]	OE is associated with invasion and brain metastasis [52]

TF, transcription factor; OE, overexpression; EMT, epithelial-mesenchymal transition. Numbers in brackets refer to the list of reference.

Table 1.
Main TSGs with dual functions reported in lung cancer.

the binding of a p53 tetramer to the promoter of target genes [25]. In many cancer types, *TP53* mutation is associated with poor prognosis, including local and distant metastases events, resistance to treatment and decreased survival [26, 27].

Despite having a reputation as a 'guardian of the genome', recent work has shown that activating *TP53* alterations can act to promote cancer development and progression [25, 28]. Depending on the location of the mutation within the *TP53* gene, protein structure and subsequent DNA binding activity can be lost or altered, resulting in either loss or gain of function [25]. In contrast to the majority of TSGs, *TP53* is not commonly inactivated by deletions or truncating mutations. Indeed, 74% of mutations within the *TP53* locus are missense point mutations, which can be found in proteins in human tumours [25]. In fact, altered *TP53* was initially considered as a cancer antigen with putative oncogenic properties [25]. Together, this highlights the dichotomous role of *TP53* disruptions, in that both the loss of wild-type p53 and gain-of-function mutations can provide a growth advantage to tumours [28].

Lung cancer is commonly associated with tobacco use, where the prolonged exposure to carcinogens damages the DNA of the exposed cells. These alterations are especially enriched in missense mutations in *TP53*, leading to GOF-p53 [29]. The oncogenic GOF mutation in p53 was previously shown to be related with the inactivation of AMP-activated protein kinase (AMPK) signalling in head and neck cancer and another tobacco-related cancer [30]. AMPK is a master regulator of metabolic homeostasis and GOF-mutated p53 is able to physically interact and inhibit AMPK, stimulating aerobic glycolysis under energetic stress conditions and leading to invasive growth.

In lung cancer mouse models, prevention of tumour formation by inhibiting GOF p53 mutants has been demonstrated [53]. Although the highly aberrant genomes in p53-mutated tumours should lead to unfeasible mitosis, these mutations facilitate the survival and proliferation of these cells through stabilizing replication forks and promoting micronuclei arrangement [31].

GOF p53 mutants are most likely involved in multiple mechanisms that coordinate tumour progression. For example, GOF-p53 (R175H, R273H and D281G) was demonstrated to upregulate *CXCL5, CXCL8* and *CXCL12* through its transcription factor activity, promoting migration of lung cancer cell lines [54]. *CXCL5* expression was shown to be elevated in human lung tumour samples harbouring GOF-p53, and its inhibition could reverse cell motility in lung cancer and melanoma cell lines [54]. In NSCLC, it was recently reported that GOF-p53 can physically interact with HIF-1 and binds to the SWI/SNF chromatin remodelling complex, inducing the expression of hypoxia-responsive genes [55]. Importantly, specific extracellular matrix components are upregulated by this process and mediate pro-tumourigenic features in NSCLC [55].

2.2 *NFIB*

Nuclear factor I (NFI) is a transcription factor family, comprising NFIA, NFIB, NFIC and NFIX, that plays important roles in normal development and in numerous diseases [56]. These proteins bind to specific DNA sequences leading to repression or activation of gene expression in a context-dependent manner, regulating cell differentiation and proliferation through their target genes [57]. *NFIB*, in particular, has been implicated in a wide range of malignancies, being described as both an oncogene and a potential TSG [58].

Using an *in vivo* model, it was demonstrated that NFIB is a metastatic driver in SCLC, inducing global chromatin reprogramming during metastasis [33]. The authors isolated tumour cells from primary and metastatic sites of genetically engineered mice, and using genome-wide analysis, they showed a pronounced increase in chromatin accessibility during tumour progression, resulting from *NFIB* copy number amplifications. Interestingly, the distal regions that became accessible upon *NFIB* upregulation were similar to open regions found in neural tissue. Recently, the same group described two metastatic models in SCLC, one dependent and other independent of *NFIB* amplification [59]. *NFIB* was likewise reported as amplified and/or overexpressed in melanoma [60], breast [61], oesophagus [62] and salivary gland malignancies [63].

A gene fusion involving *NFIB* (*MYB-NFIB*) is frequently found in adenoid cystic carcinomas from salivary glands [64] and in adenoid cystic carcinoma from other topologies [65]. Despite the putative oncogenic function of *NFIB*, studies have focused on its fusion partner *MYB* as the main oncogenic driver in these cancers [66]. Given the fact that other fusion partners of *NFIB* have been reported in adenoid cystic carcinomas [67] and that *MYB-NFIB* fusions lead to *NFIB* truncation [68], *NFIB* may have a possible independent role as a TSG in these malignancies.

While the *MYB-NFIB* fusion is not observed in lung cancers, *NFIB* is frequently underexpressed in NSCLC tissues [32] and during epithelial-to-mesenchymal transition in NSCLC cell lines [69]. NFIB is an essential transcriptional factor in lung development [70] and was demonstrated to be targeted by many microRNAs that recapitulate their foetal lung expression patterns in NSCLC [32]. Lower expression of this gene was associated with shorter overall survival, less-differentiated tumour features and repressed expression of cell differentiation markers in LUAD patients [32]. Therefore, contrary to the established oncogenic role of NFIB in SCLC, these observations suggest a tumour suppressive role in NSCLC.

2.3 *NOTCH* gene family

The Notch signalling pathway is important in the regulation of cell fate during embryogenesis and maintenance of homeostasis in adult tissues [71]. It includes Notch receptors (NOTCH1, NOTCH2, NOTCH3 and NOTCH4) and ligands from the DSL family, which suppress or induce tumour-related mechanisms under specific cellular contexts [71].

In SCLC, Notch signalling is frequently inactivated by either a mutation in Notch receptors or the overexpression of ligands that inhibit downstream signalling [34]. Despite this potential role as a TSG, Notch signalling in lung tumours is complex, as it has also been shown to be related to chemoresistance in SCLC [72]. In addition, the overactivation of this pathway through several mechanisms acts like an oncogene in LUAD by preserving stem cell features and promoting proliferation [35, 73]. Notch1 expression is required in Kras-driven LUAD carcinogenesis, suppressing apoptosis via the p53 pathway [35]. The inhibition of the Notch pathway is able to restrain lung cancer stem cell maintenance, which is characterized by subpopulations of cells expressing aldehyde dehydrogenase [74].

Conversely, loss-of-function mutations of Notch receptors generating truncated receptors imply a TSG role in LUSC [75]. Although functional studies to further corroborate this hypothesis are still needed, reports in other squamous cell carcinomas substantiate the idea that the inactivation of this signalling pathway promotes tumourigenesis [76].

2.4 *NKX2-1* (also known as *TTF-1*)

Nkx2-1 is a homeobox-containing transcription factor that is essential for lung development and is expressed in type II pneumocytes and bronchiolar cells in adults [77]. It is expressed in 40–50% of lung cancers and is amplified and overexpressed in 6–11% of LUAD [78].

Nkx2-1 acts as a lineage-specific oncogene in some LUAD cases [79], enhancing cell viability and proliferation in lung cancer cell lines [78]. This function relies on the activation of (i) the pro-survival PI3K-AKT pathway, through ROR1 kinase-dependent c-Src activation as well as maintaining the EGFR-ERBB3 association [80], and (ii) LMO3, a member of the LMO family of oncogenes that is translocated in T-ALL [81].

On the other hand, *Nkx2-1* expression has been associated with good patient outcome [82] and the loss of *Nkx2-1* expression was associated with the aggressive behaviour of NSCLCs [83]. Mechanistically, tumour suppressive functions of Nkx2-1 in lung adenocarcinoma rely on the restriction of cell motility, invasion and metastatic ability, through the inhibition of the TGF-β [41] and IKK-B/NFk-B [39] pathways. The dual role of Nkx2-1 is dependent on *EGFR, KRAS* and *TP53* status in LUAD: *NKX2-1* acts as a TSG in *KRAS*-driven and *TP53*-mutant tumours, whereas it enhances *EGFR*-driven tumourigenesis [84, 85].

2.5 *NFE2L2*

NFE2L2 encodes a transcription factor that regulates proteins involved in cellular defense mechanisms against metabolic, xenobiotic and oxidative stress [86]. *NFE2L2* has been often considered a TSG due to its protective role against genome-damaging agents, the higher propensity to cancer development in *NFE2L2*-deficient mice and its protective effects in cancer chemoprevention [87].

Due to the constant exposure to oxidative stress in the lung, the *NFE2L2* pathway is important to guarantee the genomic stability of these cells [88]. However, once transformation of normal to cancer cells occurs, *NFE2L2* favours tumour development by acting to protect against oxidative stress resulting from the tumour microenvironment and exposure to genotoxic agents during patient treatment [86]. In fact, mutations in *NFE2L2* and *KEAP1,* an important member of the *NFE2L2* signalling, are very common and mutually exclusive in NSCLC [89]. Curiously, a recent study demonstrated that lung cancer patients presenting *NFE2L2* or *KEAP1* mutations are highly resistant to chemotherapy [89]. However, the relation between the *NFE2L2* pathway and treatment response prediction needs further investigation.

2.6 *MALAT1* and other non-coding RNAs

While large-scale genomic sequencing efforts have uncovered an invaluable number of genetic alterations related to cancer biology, in the past, they were commonly focused on the 2% of the genome that encodes protein [90]. In the last decade, non-coding RNA transcripts have been shown to have important regulatory functions in normal and disease biology [91]. Indeed, many non-coding genes have been shown to play tumour-suppressive or oncogenic roles in numerous cancer types [92].

Metastasis-associated lung adenocarcinoma transcript 1 (*MALAT1*) was one of the first cancer-related long non-coding RNAs to be described [93]. *MALAT1* is broadly expressed in normal cells, where it has been shown to regulate the alternative splicing of pre-mRNAs by changing the distribution of splicing regulators in nuclear speckles [94]. *MALAT1* was primarily identified as an oncogenic transcript in lung cancer and has since been widely considered a marker of metastasis, poor patient survival [93] and chemotherapy resistance in NSCLC [48]. Mechanistically, *MALAT1* has been shown to promote carcinogenesis through P53 deacetylation [95] and enhance cell migration through Akt/mTOR signalling [96] and TGF-β-induced endothelial-to-mesenchymal transition [97]. Conversely, *MALAT1* has also been shown to reduce invasiveness by modulating the expression of EpCAM and ITGB4 in PTEN-expressing tumours [47] and by downregulation of MMP2 and inactivation of ERK/MAPK signalling [98]. *MALAT1* also binds the nuclear p65/p50 heterodimer and thus inhibits NF-κB-dependent pathways [99] and is thought to be involved in the response to DNA damage [100]. Furthermore, *MALAT1* reduces the invasiveness of cerebral metastases by sustaining the blood-brain barrier [101]. *MALAT1* expression and subcellular location is finely tuned through various regulatory mechanisms [102], which may drive its pro- or anti-tumour effects [103]. Analysis of the dual role of *MALAT1* highlights not only the complexity of non-coding RNA function but also their relevance to broad areas of cancer biology and management.

MicroRNAs (miRNAs) are short transcripts that typically regulate coding genes post-transcriptionally through direct interaction with mRNA transcripts. Many are deregulated in lung cancer [104], where they have documented tumour-suppressive and oncogenic roles [105]. For example, miRNA-125b has been shown to have a multifaceted function as a tumour suppressor and oncogene, being underexpressed in bladder [106] and ovarian cancer [107] and overexpressed in glioma [108] and prostate cancer [109]. It was shown that miRNA-125b induces apoptosis in cancer cell lines exposed to nutrient starvation and chemotherapy, including in lung cancer [49]. On the other hand, miRNA-125b may also function as an oncogene in NSCLC, as it is able to promote metastasis by targeting TP53INP1 [50]. In addition, inhibition of miR-125b can also decrease the invasive potential and leads to cell cycle arrest and apoptosis in NSCLC [110]. Similarly, miR-378 was reported to be overexpressed in lung cancer and other tumour types, inducing cell migration, invasion and tumour angiogenesis [111]. However, it was previously demonstrated that upregulation of this miRNA sensitizes lung cancer cell lines to cisplatin [51].

3. Conclusions and future directions

Here, we summarize the commonly disrupted genes in lung cancer with dual roles as both tumour suppressors and oncogenes. These conflicting roles are a result from the complexity of biological pathways and the heterogeneity of cancer cells.

Most of the current molecular therapies are based on hyperactivated oncogene inhibitors. In lung cancer, only a fraction of the cases exhibit alterations in targetable genes, such as *EGFR, BRAF* and *MET* mutations and *ALK, RET* and *ROS1* fusions [112]. Therefore, there is an urgent need for the development of novel therapeutic strategies exploiting non-oncogene alterations of lung tumour cells.

Considering that TSGs are found altered more frequently than oncogenes in human tumours [113], the existence of TSGs with dual oncogenic roles opens a new window of opportunities for the development of new targeted therapies. However, therapeutic action against TSGs remains challenging, as many are not amenable to current pharmacologic inactivation strategies. Most of the TSGs are not a kinase that can be pharmacologically blocked and are not located at the cell surface to be targeted by an antibody.

In summary, there is an unmet need to clarify the ambiguity found within genes, both coding and non-coding, with both pro- and anti-tumour functions. Broadening our understanding of these features may enable the development of novel and specific therapeutic strategies that consider both molecular and tissue contexts.

Acknowledgements

This work was supported by grants from the Canadian Institutes for Health Research (CIHR FDN-143345) and scholarships from CIHR, the BC Cancer Foundation, the Ligue nationale contre le cancer, the Fonds de Recherche en Santé

Respiratoire (appel d'offres 2018 emis en commun avec la Fondation du Souffle), the Fondation Charles Nicolle and the São Paulo Research Foundation (FAPESP 2015/17707-5 and 2018/06138-8). D.D.B.S. and E.A.M. are Vanier Canada Scholars.

Conflict of interest

The authors have no conflicts to declare.

Author details

Mateus Camargo Barros-Filho[1,2*†], Florian Guisier[1,3†], Leigha D. Rock[1,4,5†], Daiana D. Becker-Santos[1], Adam P. Sage[1], Erin A. Marshall[1] and Wan L. Lam[1]

1 Department of Integrative Oncology, British Columbia Cancer Research Centre, Vancouver, BC, Canada

2 International Research Center, A.C. Camargo Cancer Center, SP, Brazil

3 Pneumology Department, Rouen University Hospital, Rouen, France

4 Department of Cancer Control Research, British Columbia Cancer Research Centre, Vancouver, BC, Canada

5 Department of Oral and Biological Medical Sciences, Faculty of Dentistry, University of British Columbia, Vancouver, BC, Canada

*Address all correspondence to: mbarros@bccrc.ca

† These authors contributed equally to this work

References

[1] Hanahan D, Weinberg RA. Hallmarks of cancer: The next generation. Cell. 2011;**144**(5):646-674

[2] Gupta PB, Fillmore CM, Jiang G, Shapira SD, Tao K, Kuperwasser C, et al. Stochastic state transitions give rise to phenotypic equilibrium in populations of cancer cells. Cell. 2011;**146**(4):633-644

[3] Dagogo-Jack I, Shaw AT. Tumour heterogeneity and resistance to cancer therapies. Nature Reviews Clinical Oncology. 2018;**15**(2):81-94

[4] Stepanenko AA, Vassetzky YS, Kavsan VM. Antagonistic functional duality of cancer genes. Gene. 2013;**529**(2):199-207

[5] Shen L, Shi Q, Wang W. Double agents: Genes with both oncogenic and tumor-suppressor functions. Oncogene. 2018;**7**(3):25

[6] Aranko AS, Oeemig JS, Kajander T, Iwai H. Intermolecular domain swapping induces intein-mediated protein alternative splicing. Nature Chemical Biology. 2013;**9**(10):616-622

[7] Knudson AG. Two genetic hits (more or less) to cancer. Nature Reviews Cancer. 2001;**1**(2):157-162

[8] Ferlay J, Soerjomataram I, Dikshit R, Eser S, Mathers C, Rebelo M, et al. Cancer incidence and mortality worldwide: Sources, methods and major patterns in GLOBOCAN 2012. International Journal of Cancer. 2015;**136**(5):E359-E386

[9] Noone AM, Cronin KA, Altekruse SF, Howlader N, Lewis DR, Petkov VI, et al. Cancer incidence and survival trends by subtype using data from the surveillance epidemiology and end results program, 1992-2013. Cancer Epidemiology, Biomarkers & Prevention. 2017;**26**(4):632-641

[10] Ridge CA, McErlean AM, Ginsberg MS. Epidemiology of lung cancer. Seminars in Interventional Radiology. 2013;**30**(2):93-98

[11] Thun MJ, Hannan LM, Adams-Campbell LL, Boffetta P, Buring JE, Feskanich D, et al. Lung cancer occurrence in never-smokers: An analysis of 13 cohorts and 22 cancer registry studies. PLoS Medicine. 2008;**5**(9):e185

[12] Dela Cruz CS, Tanoue LT, Matthay RA. Lung cancer: Epidemiology, etiology, and prevention. Clinics in Chest Medicine. 2011;**32**(4):605-644

[13] Pikor LA, Ramnarine VR, Lam S, Lam WL. Genetic alterations defining NSCLC subtypes and their therapeutic implications. Lung Cancer. 2013;**82**(2):179-189

[14] Gazdar AF, Bunn PA, Minna JD. Small-cell lung cancer: What we know, what we need to know and the path forward. Nature Reviews Cancer. 2017;**17**(12):725-737

[15] Chen Z, Fillmore CM, Hammerman PS, Kim CF, Wong KK. Non-small-cell lung cancers: A heterogeneous set of diseases. Nature Reviews Cancer. 2014;**14**(8):535-546

[16] George J, Lim JS, Jang SJ, Cun Y, Ozretic L, Kong G, et al. Comprehensive genomic profiles of small cell lung cancer. Nature. 2015;**524**(7563):47-53

[17] Lockwood WW, Wilson IM, Coe BP, Chari R, Pikor LA, Thu KL, et al. Divergent genomic and epigenomic landscapes of lung cancer subtypes underscore the selection of different oncogenic pathways during tumor development. PLoS One. 2012;**7**(5):e37775

[18] Heath EI, Lynce F, Xiu J, Ellerbrock A, Reddy SK, Obeid E, et al. Racial

disparities in the molecular landscape of cancer. Anticancer Research. 2018;**38**(4):2235-2240

[19] Govindan R, Ding L, Griffith M, Subramanian J, Dees ND, Kanchi KL, et al. Genomic landscape of non-small cell lung cancer in smokers and never-smokers. Cell. 2012;**150**(6):1121-1134

[20] Zhu CQ, Cutz JC, Liu N, Lau D, Shepherd FA, Squire JA, et al. Amplification of telomerase (hTERT) gene is a poor prognostic marker in non-small-cell lung cancer. British Journal of Cancer. 2006;**94**(10):1452-1459

[21] Shi J, Hua X, Zhu B, Ravichandran S, Wang M, Nguyen C, et al. Somatic genomics and clinical features of lung adenocarcinoma: A retrospective study. PLoS Medicine. 2016;**13**(12):e1002162

[22] Barlesi F, Mazieres J, Merlio JP, Debieuvre D, Mosser J, Lena H, et al. Routine molecular profiling of patients with advanced non-small-cell lung cancer: Results of a 1-year nationwide programme of the French Cooperative Thoracic Intergroup (IFCT). Lancet. 2016;**387**(10026):1415-1426

[23] Campbell JD, Alexandrov A, Kim J, Wala J, Berger AH, Pedamallu CS, et al. Distinct patterns of somatic genome alterations in lung adenocarcinomas and squamous cell carcinomas. Nature Genetics. 2016;**48**(6):607-616

[24] Bailey MH, Tokheim C, Porta-Pardo E, Sengupta S, Bertrand D, Weerasinghe A, et al. Comprehensive characterization of cancer driver genes and mutations. Cell. 2018;**173**(2):371-385.e18

[25] Brosh R, Rotter V. When mutants gain new powers: News from the mutant p53 field. Nature Reviews Cancer. 2009;**9**(10):701-713

[26] Campling BG, El-Deiry WS. Clinical implication of p53 mutation in lung cancer. Molecular Biotechnology. 2003;**24**(2):141-156

[27] Zhou G, Liu Z, Myers JN. TP53 mutations in head and neck squamous cell carcinoma and their impact on disease progression and treatment response. Journal of Cellular Biochemistry. 2016;**117**(12):2682-2692

[28] Soussi T, Wiman KG. TP53: An oncogene in disguise. Cell Death and Differentiation. 2015;**22**(8):1239-1249

[29] Barta JA, McMahon SB. Lung-enriched mutations in the p53 tumor suppressor: A paradigm for tissue-specific gain of oncogenic function. Molecular Cancer Research. 2019;**17**(1):3-9

[30] Zhou G, Wang J, Zhao M, Xie TX, Tanaka N, Sano D, et al. Gain-of-function mutant p53 promotes cell growth and cancer cell metabolism via inhibition of AMPK activation. Molecular Cell. 2014;**54**(6):960-974

[31] Singh S, Vaughan CA, Frum RA, Grossman SR, Deb S, Palit DS. Mutant p53 establishes targetable tumor dependency by promoting unscheduled replication. The Journal of Clinical Investigation. 2017;**127**(5):1839-1855

[32] Becker-Santos DD, Thu KL, English JC, Pikor LA, Martinez VD, Zhang M, et al. Developmental transcription factor NFIB is a putative target of oncofetal miRNAs and is associated with tumour aggressiveness in lung adenocarcinoma. The Journal of Pathology. 2016;**240**(2):161-172

[33] Denny SK, Yang D, Chuang CH, Brady JJ, Lim JS, Gruner BM, et al. Nfib promotes metastasis through a widespread increase in chromatin accessibility. Cell. 2016;**166**(2):328-342

[34] Meder L, Konig K, Ozretic L, Schultheis AM, Ueckeroth F, Ade CP, et al. NOTCH, ASCL1, p53 and RB

alterations define an alternative pathway driving neuroendocrine and small cell lung carcinomas. International Journal of Cancer. 2016;**138**(4):927-938

[35] Licciulli S, Avila JL, Hanlon L, Troutman S, Cesaroni M, Kota S, et al. Notch1 is required for Kras-induced lung adenocarcinoma and controls tumor cell survival via p53. Cancer Research. 2013;**73**(19):5974-5984

[36] Tong YH, Zhang B, Fan Y, Lin NM. Keap1-Nrf2 pathway: A promising target towards lung cancer prevention and therapeutics. Chronic Diseases and Translational Medicine. 2015;**1**(3):175-186

[37] Menegon S, Columbano A, Giordano S. The dual roles of NRF2 in cancer. Trends in Molecular Medicine. 2016;**22**(7):578-593

[38] Winslow MM, Dayton TL, Verhaak RG, Kim-Kiselak C, Snyder EL, Feldser DM, et al. Suppression of lung adenocarcinoma progression by Nkx2-1. Nature. 2011;**473**(7345):101-104

[39] Chen PM, Wu TC, Cheng YW, Chen CY, Lee H. NKX2-1-mediated p53 expression modulates lung adenocarcinoma progression via modulating IKKbeta/NF-kappaB activation. Oncotarget. 2015;**6**(16):14274-14289

[40] Kottakis F, Bardeesy N. LKB1-AMPK axis revisited. Cell Research. 2012;**22**(12):1617-1620

[41] Saito RA, Watabe T, Horiguchi K, Kohyama T, Saitoh M, Nagase T, et al. Thyroid transcription factor-1 inhibits transforming growth factor-beta-mediated epithelial-to-mesenchymal transition in lung adenocarcinoma cells. Cancer Research. 2009;**69**(7):2783-2791

[42] Pirozzi G, Tirino V, Camerlingo R, Franco R, La Rocca A, Liguori E, et al. Epithelial to mesenchymal transition by TGFbeta-1 induction increases stemness characteristics in primary non small cell lung cancer cell line. PLoS One. 2011;**6**(6):e21548

[43] Peng Y, Cao J, Yao XY, Wang JX, Zhong MZ, Gan PP, et al. TUSC3 induces autophagy in human non-small cell lung cancer cells through Wnt/beta-catenin signaling. Oncotarget. 2017;**8**(32):52960-52974

[44] Feng S, Zhai J, Lu D, Lin J, Dong X, Liu X, et al. TUSC3 accelerates cancer growth and induces epithelial-mesenchymal transition by upregulating claudin-1 in non-small-cell lung cancer cells. Experimental Cell Research. 2018;**373**(1-2):44-56

[45] Huff V. Wilms' tumours: About tumour suppressor genes, an oncogene and a chameleon gene. Nature Reviews Cancer. 2011;**11**(2):111-121

[46] Wu C, Wang S, Xu C, Tyler A, Li X, Andersson C, et al. WT1 enhances proliferation and impedes apoptosis in KRAS mutant NSCLC via targeting cMyc. Cellular Physiology and Biochemistry. 2015;**35**(2):647-662

[47] Kwok ZH, Roche V, Chew XH, Fadieieva A, Tay Y. A non-canonical tumor suppressive role for the long non-coding RNA MALAT1 in colon and breast cancers. International Journal of Cancer. 2018;**143**(3):668-678

[48] Cui Y, Li G, Zhang X, Dai F, Zhang R. Increased MALAT1 expression contributes to cisplatin resistance in non-small cell lung cancer. Oncology Letters. 2018;**16**(4):4821-4828

[49] Gong J, Zhang JP, Li B, Zeng C, You K, Chen MX, et al. MicroRNA-125b promotes apoptosis by regulating the expression of Mcl-1, Bcl-w and IL-6R. Oncogene. 2013;**32**(25):3071-3079

[50] Li Q, Han Y, Wang C, Shan S, Wang Y, Zhang J, et al. MicroRNA-125b

promotes tumor metastasis through targeting tumor protein 53-induced nuclear protein 1 in patients with non-small-cell lung cancer. Cancer Cell International. 2015;**15**:84

[51] Chen X, Jiang Y, Huang Z, Li D, Cao M, Meng Q, et al. miRNA-378 reverses chemoresistance to cisplatin in lung adenocarcinoma cells by targeting secreted clusterin. Scientific Reports. 2016;**6**:19455

[52] Chen LT, Xu SD, Xu H, Zhang JF, Ning JF, Wang SF. MicroRNA-378 is associated with non-small cell lung cancer brain metastasis by promoting cell migration, invasion and tumor angiogenesis. Medical Oncology. 2012;**29**(3):1673-1680

[53] Vaughan CA, Singh S, Windle B, Sankala HM, Graves PR, Andrew Yeudall W, et al. p53 mutants induce transcription of NF-kappaB2 in H1299 cells through CBP and STAT binding on the NF-kappaB2 promoter and gain of function activity. Archives of Biochemistry and Biophysics. 2012;**518**(1):79-88

[54] Yeudall WA, Vaughan CA, Miyazaki H, Ramamoorthy M, Choi MY, Chapman CG, et al. Gain-of-function mutant p53 upregulates CXC chemokines and enhances cell migration. Carcinogenesis. 2012;**33**(2):442-451

[55] Amelio I, Mancini M, Petrova V, Cairns RA, Vikhreva P, Nicolai S, et al. p53 mutants cooperate with HIF-1 in transcriptional regulation of extracellular matrix components to promote tumor progression. Proceedings of the National Academy of Sciences of the United States of America. 2018;**115**(46):e10869-e10878

[56] Mason S, Piper M, Gronostajski RM, Richards LJ. Nuclear factor one transcription factors in CNS development. Molecular Neurobiology. 2009;**39**(1):10-23

[57] Gronostajski RM. Roles of the NFI/CTF gene family in transcription and development. Gene. 2000;**249**(1-2):31-45

[58] Becker-Santos DD, Lonergan KM, Gronostajski RM, Lam WL. Nuclear factor I/B: A master regulator of cell differentiation with paradoxical roles in cancer. eBioMedicine. 2017;**22**:2-9

[59] Yang D, Denny SK, Greenside PG, Chaikovsky AC, Brady JJ, Ouadah Y, et al. Intertumoral heterogeneity in SCLC is influenced by the cell type of origin. Cancer Discovery. 2018;**8**(10):1316-1331

[60] Fane ME, Chhabra Y, Hollingsworth DEJ, Simmons JL, Spoerri L, Oh TG, et al. NFIB mediates BRN2 driven melanoma cell migration and invasion through regulation of EZH2 and MITF. eBioMedicine. 2017;**16**:63-75

[61] Moon HG, Hwang KT, Kim JA, Kim HS, Lee MJ, Jung EM, et al. NFIB is a potential target for estrogen receptor-negative breast cancers. Molecular Oncology. 2011;**5**(6):538-544

[62] Yang ZQ, Imoto I, Pimkhaokham A, Shimada Y, Sasaki K, Oka M, et al. A novel amplicon at 9p23-24 in squamous cell carcinoma of the esophagus that lies proximal to GASC1 and harbors NFIB. Japanese Journal of Cancer Research. 2001;**92**(4):423-428

[63] Andreasen S, Persson M, Kiss K, Homoe P, Heegaard S, Stenman G. Genomic profiling of a combined large cell neuroendocrine carcinoma of the submandibular gland. Oncology Reports. 2016;**35**(4):2177-2182

[64] Warner KA, Oklejas AE, Pearson AT, Zhang Z, Wu W, Divi V, et al. UM-HACC-2A: MYB-NFIB fusion-positive human adenoid cystic

carcinoma cell line. Oral Oncology. 2018;**87**:21-28

[65] Brill LB 2nd, Kanner WA, Fehr A, Andren Y, Moskaluk CA, Loning T, et al. Analysis of MYB expression and MYB-NFIB gene fusions in adenoid cystic carcinoma and other salivary neoplasms. Modern Pathology. 2011;**24**(9):1169-1176

[66] Persson M, Andren Y, Mark J, Horlings HM, Persson F, Stenman G. Recurrent fusion of MYB and NFIB transcription factor genes in carcinomas of the breast and head and neck. Proceedings of the National Academy of Sciences of the United States of America. 2009;**106**(44):18740-18744

[67] Geurts JM, Schoenmakers EF, Roijer E, Astrom AK, Stenman G, van de Ven WJ. Identification of NFIB as recurrent translocation partner gene of HMGIC in pleomorphic adenomas. Oncogene. 1998;**16**(7):865-872

[68] Ho AS, Kannan K, Roy DM, Morris LG, Ganly I, Katabi N, et al. The mutational landscape of adenoid cystic carcinoma. Nature Genetics. 2013;**45**(7):791-798

[69] Du L, Yamamoto S, Burnette BL, Huang D, Gao K, Jamshidi N, et al. Transcriptome profiling reveals novel gene expression signatures and regulating transcription factors of TGFbeta-induced epithelial-to-mesenchymal transition. Cancer Medicine. 2016;**5**(8):1962-1972

[70] Steele-Perkins G, Plachez C, Butz KG, Yang G, Bachurski CJ, Kinsman SL, et al. The transcription factor gene Nfib is essential for both lung maturation and brain development. Molecular and Cellular Biology. 2005;**25**(2):685-698

[71] Hori K, Sen A, Artavanis-Tsakonas S. Notch signaling at a glance. Journal of Cell Science. 2013;**126**(Pt 10): 2135-2140

[72] Lim JS, Ibaseta A, Fischer MM, Cancilla B, O'Young G, Cristea S, et al. Intratumoural heterogeneity generated by Notch signalling promotes small-cell lung cancer. Nature. 2017;**545**(7654):360-364

[73] Ntziachristos P, Lim JS, Sage J, Aifantis I. From fly wings to targeted cancer therapies: A centennial for notch signaling. Cancer Cell. 2014;**25**(3):318-334

[74] Sullivan JP, Spinola M, Dodge M, Raso MG, Behrens C, Gao B, et al. Aldehyde dehydrogenase activity selects for lung adenocarcinoma stem cells dependent on notch signaling. Cancer Research. 2010;**70**(23):9937-9948

[75] Wang NJ, Sanborn Z, Arnett KL, Bayston LJ, Liao W, Proby CM, et al. Loss-of-function mutations in Notch receptors in cutaneous and lung squamous cell carcinoma. Proceedings of the National Academy of Sciences of the United States of America. 2011;**108**(43):17761-17766

[76] Zhang M, Biswas S, Qin X, Gong W, Deng W, Yu H. Does Notch play a tumor suppressor role across diverse squamous cell carcinomas? Cancer Medicine. 2016;**5**(8):2048-2060

[77] Maeda Y, Dave V, Whitsett JA. Transcriptional control of lung morphogenesis. Physiological Reviews. 2007;**87**(1):219-244

[78] Kwei KA, Kim YH, Girard L, Kao J, Pacyna-Gengelbach M, Salari K, et al. Genomic profiling identifies TITF1 as a lineage-specific oncogene amplified in lung cancer. Oncogene. 2008;**27**(25):3635-3640

[79] Yamaguchi T, Hosono Y, Yanagisawa K, Takahashi T. NKX2-1/TTF-1: An enigmatic oncogene that functions as a double-edged sword for cancer cell survival and progression. Cancer Cell. 2013;**23**(6):718-723

[80] Yamaguchi T, Yanagisawa K, Sugiyama R, Hosono Y, Shimada Y, Arima C, et al. NKX2-1/TITF1/TTF-1-induced ROR1 is required to sustain EGFR survival signaling in lung adenocarcinoma. Cancer Cell. 2012;**21**(3):348-361

[81] Watanabe H, Francis JM, Woo MS, Etemad B, Lin W, Fries DF, et al. Integrated cistromic and expression analysis of amplified NKX2-1 in lung adenocarcinoma identifies LMO3 as a functional transcriptional target. Genes & Development. 2013;**27**(2):197-210

[82] Berghmans T, Paesmans M, Mascaux C, Martin B, Meert AP, Haller A, et al. Thyroid transcription factor 1-a new prognostic factor in lung cancer: A meta-analysis. Annals of Oncology. 2006;**17**(11):1673-1676

[83] Tan D, Li Q, Deeb G, Ramnath N, Slocum HK, Brooks J, et al. Thyroid transcription factor-1 expression prevalence and its clinical implications in non-small cell lung cancer: A high-throughput tissue microarray and immunohistochemistry study. Human Pathology. 2003;**34**(6):597-604

[84] Maeda Y, Tsuchiya T, Hao H, Tompkins DH, Xu Y, Mucenski ML, et al. Kras(G12D) and Nkx2-1 haploinsufficiency induce mucinous adenocarcinoma of the lung. The Journal of Clinical Investigation. 2012;**122**(12):4388-4400

[85] Snyder EL, Watanabe H, Magendantz M, Hoersch S, Chen TA, Wang DG, et al. Nkx2-1 represses a latent gastric differentiation program in lung adenocarcinoma. Molecular Cell. 2013;**50**(2):185-199

[86] Motohashi H, Yamamoto M. Nrf2-Keap1 defines a physiologically important stress response mechanism. Trends in Molecular Medicine. 2004;**10**(11):549-557

[87] Hayes JD, McMahon M, Chowdhry S, Dinkova-Kostova AT. Cancer chemoprevention mechanisms mediated through the Keap1-Nrf2 pathway. Antioxidants & Redox Signaling. 2010;**13**(11):1713-1748

[88] Siegel D, Franklin WA, Ross D. Immunohistochemical detection of NAD(P)H:quinone oxidoreductase in human lung and lung tumors. Clinical Cancer Research. 1998;**4**(9):2065-2070

[89] Frank R, Scheffler M, Merkelbach-Bruse S, Ihle MA, Kron A, Rauer M, et al. Clinical and pathological characteristics of KEAP1- and NFE2L2-mutated non-small cell lung carcinoma (NSCLC). Clinical Cancer Research. 2018;**24**(13):3087-3096

[90] Carninci P, Kasukawa T, Katayama S, Gough J, Frith MC, Maeda N, et al. The transcriptional landscape of the mammalian genome. Science. 2005;**309**(5740):1559-1563

[91] Esteller M. Non-coding RNAs in human disease. Nature Reviews Genetics. 2011;**12**(12):861-874

[92] Zhang W, Bojorquez-Gomez A, Velez DO, Xu G, Sanchez KS, Shen JP, et al. A global transcriptional network connecting noncoding mutations to changes in tumor gene expression. Nature Genetics. 2018;**50**(4):613-620

[93] Ji P, Diederichs S, Wang W, Boing S, Metzger R, Schneider PM, et al. MALAT-1, a novel noncoding RNA, and thymosin beta4 predict metastasis and survival in early-stage non-small cell lung cancer. Oncogene. 2003;**22**(39):8031-8041

[94] Tripathi V, Ellis JD, Shen Z, Song DY, Pan Q, Watt AT, et al. The nuclear-retained noncoding RNA MALAT1 regulates alternative splicing by modulating SR splicing factor phosphorylation. Molecular Cell. 2010;**39**(6):925-938

[95] Chen R, Liu Y, Zhuang H, Yang B, Hei K, Xiao M, et al. Quantitative proteomics reveals that long non-coding RNA MALAT1 interacts with DBC1 to regulate p53 acetylation. Nucleic Acids Research. 2017;**45**(17):9947-9959

[96] Tang Y, Xiao G, Chen Y, Deng Y. LncRNA MALAT1 promotes migration and invasion of non-small-cell lung cancer by targeting miR-206 and activating Akt/mTOR signaling. Anti-Cancer Drugs. 2018;**29**(8):725-735

[97] Xiang Y, Zhang Y, Tang Y, Li Q. MALAT1 modulates TGF-beta1-induced endothelial-to-mesenchymal transition through downregulation of miR-145. Cellular Physiology and Biochemistry. 2017;**42**(1):357-372

[98] Han Y, Wu Z, Wu T, Huang Y, Cheng Z, Li X, et al. Tumor-suppressive function of long noncoding RNA MALAT1 in glioma cells by downregulation of MMP2 and inactivation of ERK/MAPK signaling. Cell Death & Disease. 2016;7:e2123

[99] Zhao G, Su Z, Song D, Mao Y, Mao X. The long noncoding RNA MALAT1 regulates the lipopolysaccharide-induced inflammatory response through its interaction with NF-kappaB. FEBS Letters. 2016;**590**(17):2884-2895

[100] Gao C, He Z, Li J, Li X, Bai Q, Zhang Z, et al. Specific long non-coding RNAs response to occupational PAHs exposure in coke oven workers. Toxicology Reports. 2016;**3**:160-166

[101] Ma J, Wang P, Yao Y, Liu Y, Li Z, Liu X, et al. Knockdown of long non-coding RNA MALAT1 increases the blood-tumor barrier permeability by up-regulating miR-140. Biochimica et Biophysica Acta. 2016;**1859**(2):324-338

[102] Gutschner T, Hammerle M, Diederichs S. MALAT1—A paradigm for long noncoding RNA function in cancer. Journal of Molecular Medicine. 2013;**91**(7):791-801

[103] Guo F, Guo L, Li Y, Zhou Q, Li Z. MALAT1 is an oncogenic long non-coding RNA associated with tumor invasion in non-small cell lung cancer regulated by DNA methylation. International Journal of Clinical and Experimental Pathology. 2015;**8**(12):15903-15910

[104] Cinegaglia NC, Andrade SC, Tokar T, Pinheiro M, Severino FE, Oliveira RA, et al. Integrative transcriptome analysis identifies deregulated microRNA-transcription factor networks in lung adenocarcinoma. Oncotarget. 2016;**7**(20):28920-28934

[105] Svoronos AA, Engelman DM, Slack FJ. OncomiR or tumor suppressor? The duplicity of micrornas in cancer. Cancer Research. 2016;**76**(13):3666-3670

[106] Ichimi T, Enokida H, Okuno Y, Kunimoto R, Chiyomaru T, Kawamoto K, et al. Identification of novel microRNA targets based on microRNA signatures in bladder cancer. International Journal of Cancer. 2009;**125**(2):345-352

[107] Guan Y, Yao H, Zheng Z, Qiu G, Sun K. MiR-125b targets BCL3 and suppresses ovarian cancer proliferation. International Journal of Cancer. 2011;**128**(10):2274-2283

[108] Pogue AI, Cui JG, Li YY, Zhao Y, Culicchia F, Lukiw WJ. Micro RNA-125b (miRNA-125b) function in astrogliosis and glial cell proliferation. Neuroscience Letters. 2010;**476**(1):18-22

[109] Ozen M, Creighton CJ, Ozdemir M, Ittmann M. Widespread deregulation of microRNA expression in human prostate cancer. Oncogene. 2008;**27**(12):1788-1793

[110] Wang X, Zhang Y, Fu Y, Zhang J, Yin L, Pu Y, et al. MicroRNA-125b may

function as an oncogene in lung cancer cells. Molecular Medicine Reports. 2015;**11**(5):3880-3887

[111] Ho CS, Yap SH, Phuah NH, In LL, Hasima N. MicroRNAs associated with tumour migration, invasion and angiogenic properties in A549 and SK-Lu1 human lung adenocarcinoma cells. Lung Cancer. 2014;**83**(2):154-162

[112] Cancer Genome Atlas Research Network. Comprehensive molecular profiling of lung adenocarcinoma. Nature. 2014;**511**(7511):543-550

[113] Vogelstein B, Papadopoulos N, Velculescu VE, Zhou S, Diaz LA Jr, Kinzler KW. Cancer genome landscapes. Science. 2013;**339**(6127):1546-1558

Chapter 4

Duplicitous Dispositions of Micro-RNAs (miRs) in Breast Cancer

Amal Qattan

Abstract

In 1993, a gene silencer known as lin-4 was first discovered in *Caenorhabditis elegans* and demonstrated to be critical for larval development. Lin-4 belongs to a family of signaling molecules known as non-protein coding microRNAs (miRNAs) which are not only highly conserved in humans, but also involved in the fundamental processes of oncogenesis. While miRNAs are not translated to proteins themselves, they are capable of regulating the expression and translation of other genes thus affecting a multitude of biological and pathological pathways as well as those essential to the malignant landscape. The aim of this chapter is to explore the diverse roles of miRNAs in the context of breast cancer. Following a brief overview of miRNA biogenesis, this chapter covers the production of miRNAs by tumor cells and stromal cells, onco-suppressor miRNAs, use as therapeutics, contribution to therapeutic resistance, and finally their emerging role as biomarkers.

Keywords: microRNAs (miRs), breast cancer epigenetic alteration, microRNA-based therapy, miRNA pharmacogenomics, miRSNPs, miR-polymorphisms, clinical trials

1. Introduction

A gene silencer known as *lin-4* was first discovered in *Caenorhabditis elegans* and demonstrated to be critical for larval development [1]. *Lin-4* belongs to a family of signaling molecules known as non-protein coding microRNA (miRNAs) which are not only highly conserved in humans, but also involved in the fundamental processes of oncogenesis [2]. Approximately 2000 miRNAs are present in the human genome [3]. While miRNAs are not translated into proteins themselves, they are implicated in the regulation of 30% of all genes and are thereby capable of regulating the expression and translation of other genes influencing a multitude of biological and pathological pathways [4]. This chapter explores the diverse roles of miRNAs in the most frequent cancer among women in the world: breast cancer (BC). BC impacts 2.1 million women yearly [5] and it also causes the greatest number of cancer-related deaths among women. Early detection and diagnosis are critical to survival. In the context of BC, miRNAs are dynamically regulated implicating their use in diagnosis, prognosis and tracking of drug efficacy during treatment. Following a brief overview of miRNA biogenesis, this chapter covers the production of miRNAs by tumor cells, onco-suppressor and tumor-suppressor miRNAs, their contribution to therapeutic resistance, therapeutic miRNAs (as well as therapeutics targeting of miRNAs), and finally their emerging role as biomarkers for BC prognosis, treatment responsiveness and efficacy.

2. MiRNA biogenesis and mechanisms of action

Since 1993, researchers have proceeded to learn that miRNAs were of ancient evolutionary origins. Single stranded, non-protein coding miRNAs with genetic suppression activities were found in algae, plants, invertebrates, vertebrates and even viruses [6]. Further characterization has revealed that miRNAs are not only critical for normal human development, but their aberrant expression is associated with diseases such as cancer [7, 8].

The miRNAs are encoded by genetic sequences which may be located within the introns of protein coding genes as well as in the exons and introns of long noncoding RNAs, and even intergenic regions [9]. According to the miRIAD database, 1157 (61.5%) miRNAs are intragenic (169 exonic and 988 intronic) and 724 (38.5%) are intergenic [10]. MiRNA's are single-stranded RNA transcripts that are transcribed from DNA sequences and are usually around 22 nucleotides in length. They often form distinct secondary folding conformational motifs. Most miRNAs are first transcribed into primary miRNAs (pri-miRNAs) and processed into precursor miRNAs (pre-miRNAs) and mature miRNAs. Usually they bind to the 3′-untranslated region (UTR) of target mRNAs to suppress their target's expression by inhibiting its translation. However, they can also interact with coding sequences, the 5′UTR and gene promoter regions. Though less common, some are involved in the translation activation and stabilization of target transcripts. Furthermore, the shuttling of miRNAs between different cellular compartments can also control rates of transcription and translation of their targets.

In the canonical pathway of miRNA biogenesis, RNA polymerase II transcribes miRNAs into primary miRNAs (pri-miRNAs) greater than 200 nucleotides long. Pri-mRNAs are then cleaved into pre-mRNAs by the RNAse III enzyme, Drosha with the help of double stranded RNA binding proteins Pasha and DiGeorge Syndrome Critical Region 8 (DGCR8). The 60–70 nucleotides long pre-mRNAs are then exported out of the nucleus and into the cell cytoplasm by exportin-5 and Ran GTPase. Once in the cytoplasm, pre-mRNAs are cleaved by the RNAse III enzyme Dicer which removes hairpin loops resulting in miRNA duplexes composed of a guide strand and a passenger strand. The passenger strand is discarded and the guide strand associates with Argonaute 2 (Ago2) to form the RNA-induced silencing complex (RISC) which brings the miRNA to its target mRNA. A 6–8 nucleotide sequence on the miRNA, referred to as the "seed sequence" locates the corresponding sequence of the target mRNA. A double stranded complex is formed which impedes the ribosome from translating the target [11]. Imperfect complementarity between the seed sequence and the target mRNA can also cause target degradation indirectly via deadenylation at the 3′-UTR. Non-canonical miRNA biogenesis is less common and can generally be grouped into Drosha/DGCR8-independent and Dicer-independent pathways which are outside the scope of this chapter. In addition to the inhibition of target miRNAs, there is evidence indicating that some miRNAs directly increase target translation via recruitment of protein synthesis complexes to the translation initiation region. Alternatively, target mRNA expression can also be increased due to inhibition of modulating repressors that block translation. Moreover, some miRNAs enhance ribosome biogenesis resulting in increased protein synthesis [12].

In summary, miRNA biogenesis is a multi-step process that requires various enzymes and shuttling proteins to reach a final product. Mature miRNAs are either stable molecules with half-lives of greater than 24 h or they display shorter half-lives of less than 12 h, depending on the functionality of the product [13]. More on the regulation of miRNA expression is discussed in the next section.

3. Regulation of miRNA expression

In general, just as protein-coding genes are regulated by transcription factors (TF), TFs are one of the central ways by which miRNA expression is regulated. Tissue and developmental stage specific TFs can control the transcription of miRNA genes. Many miRNAs and TFs form autoregulatory loops, in which they mutually regulate each other [14]. In addition, various physiological and pathological stimuli, such as steroid hormones, retinoids, hypoxia, interferons, stress, as well as estrogen, can affect miRNA expression [15]. Finally, while transcription regulates the magnitude of miRNA expression, decay rates influence miRNA dynamic regulation. Slow decay leads to a high level of accumulation while fast decay leads quick changes in miRNA expression levels implying that fast turnover may be involved in transient biological processes.

Epigenetic mechanisms are heritable changes in gene expression that occur without any modifications in the DNA sequence itself and include DNA methylation and histone modifications as well as miRNAs themselves [16]. The covalent binding of methyl groups to cytosine bases located among CpG dinucleotide sequences is the major modification of eukaryotic genomes which results in down regulation of gene expression. DNA methylation controls embryonic cell fate lineages and prevents reversion to an undifferentiated state [17]. Frequency of methylation is nearly one order of magnitude higher in human miRNA genes compared to the methylation of other protein-coding genes [18, 19]. This indicates strict epigenetic control of miRNA expression and also reveals how epigenetic changes in cancer cells can lead to dysregulated expression of miRNAs by cancer cells.

Genome variations include genetic mutations and polymorphisms; defined as a DNA variation in which a possible sequence is present in at least 1% of people. Single nucleotide polymorphisms (SNPs) constitute approximately 1% of the human genome. SNPs contribute to phenotypic diversity within a species as well as disease susceptibility. MiRSNPs/miR-polymorphisms are a new mechanism and novel class of functional SNPs. As miRNA molecular interactions with their targets are affected via base pairing as well as genetic variation, such as changes in genome sequence; which influences binding energy and annealing strength, SNPs can result in no change, off target or absence of miRNA binding to the predicted target [20]. Carcinogens such as those from cigarettes, dietary elements and other foreign chemical toxicities referred to as "xenobiotics," can also affect miRNA expression. Importantly, many more changes in miRNA expression were observed in cancer-target tissues than in the non-target tissues following acute or chronic exposure to carcinogens thus implicating their use as potential biomarkers for exposure to xenobiotics [21]. Finally, circadian rhythm control of miRNA expression has significant consequences for circadian timing as some miRNAs have promoter sequences inducible by circadian clock proteins. Moreover, some miRNAs can even be regulated by light and dark cycles which confer important rhythmic expressions in organs such as the liver and heart [22].

In summary, miRNA regulation is similar to other protein coding gene regulation as changes in expression can occur based on the presences or exposure to TFs, genetic polymorphisms, epigenetic factors, xenobiotics and carcinogens. How miRNA expression is regulated in the context of BC is discussed in the next section.

4. miRNAs (miRs) production by breast cancer cells

As summarized above, TF, SNPs, epigenetics, hormones and xenobiotics all affect the regulation of miRNAs; therefore, it is not surprising that breast cancer

(BC) leads to significant, dynamic changes in miRNA expression both by tumor cells and by surrounding stromal cells. This section describes BC tumor cell production of miRNAs as well as the surrounding non-cancerous stromal cells. In general, miRNAs either support or suppress tumorigenesis and are often dysregulated due to tumor-specific epigenetic changes. Likewise, tumor secreted factors such as exosomes and cytokines can also lead to aberrant signaling in the surrounding stromal cells. Furthermore, while all BCs begin in the breast, there are many subtypes which are named to reflect their particular molecular pathogenesis. Subtype diagnosis can help select appropriate therapies. Likewise, aberrant regulation of miRNAs can be subtype specific. Therefore, this section begins with a brief overview of cancer subtypes.

Breast carcinoma can begin either in the ducts or the lobules and as such, termed either ductal carcinoma in situ (DCIS), or lobular carcinoma in situ (LCIS). Both can either stay contained to the area or travel to surrounding tissue and lymph nodes in which case the clinical diagnosis is either invasive ductal carcinoma (IDC) or invasive lobular carcinoma (ILC). IDC is the most common type of BC (50–75%) followed by ILC (5–15%) [23]. Rare BC is characterized by tumor origination in the mucinous, papillary, medullary or cribriform compartments of the breast [24]. Metastasis of breast cancer to other organs is the main cause of mortality and up to 5% of patients will already have experienced metastasis at the time of diagnosis [25].

MiRNA microarray performed on 1542 breast tissue samples procured via the Molecular Taxonomy of Breast Cancer International Consortium and the Akershus University Hospital (AHUS) revealed that no miRNAs were differentially expressed in DCIS patients relative to IDC, supporting the idea that miRNA dysregulation occurs at an early stage of BC development [26]. Among the invasive subtypes, however, expression of seven miRNAs was consistently downregulated, including tumor suppressors let-7c-5p, miR-125b-5p, miR140-3p, miR-145-3p, miR-145-5p, miR-193a-5p, and miR378a-3p while expression of four oncogenic miRNAs was consistently upregulated including miR-106b-5p, miR-142, miR-342-3p, and miR425-5p. Taken together these miRNAs may significantly contribute to the transition to an invasive BC subtype [26].

While Bloom and Richardson's histologic grading system which was modified by Elston and Ellis in 1991 is the most commonly used system to gain prognostic insight, hormone receptors status, tumor size, nodal status and whether tumorous cells have invaded the lymph or blood vessels is also considered during initial diagnosis. Hormone receptor statuses including estrogen receptor (ER) and progesterone receptor (PR) as well as the tyrosine kinase receptor, human epidermal growth receptor type two (HER2) are always measured on newly diagnosed invasive BCs. Subtypes are identified via immunohistochemical staining for hormone receptors, HER2 expression status, and Ki-67 proliferation index as: luminal A (ER-positive and/or PR-positive, HER2-negative, low proliferation), luminal B (ER-positive and/or PR-positive, HER2-negative, high proliferation; or hormone receptor (HR)-positive and HER2-positive), HER2-positive (HR-negative and HER2-positive) and finally TNBC type (HR-negative and HER2-negative) [27]. ER+ breast cancer subtype is particularly prevalent in postmenopausal women taking hormone replacement therapy (HRT) which activates the transcription factor estrogen receptor alpha (ERα) which promotes the expression of numerous oncogenic genes. While ERα-signaling is targeted by miRNAs for degradation, aberrant activation of this receptor leads to aberrant expression of miRNAs controlled by ERα-signaling [28].

Several miRNAs are both tissue and cancer specific. As the primary role of miRNA is to decrease target mRNA expression, miRNAs that are upregulated by cancerous cells are often those that support cancer growth and are referred to as oncomiRs. miR-10b, miR-21 and miR-155 are well characterized oncomiRs in BC [29]. Their main role is to downregulate tumor suppressor genes which results in the promotion of cancer cell proliferation, de-differentiation and invasion [30]. BC cells also produce less tumor-suppressor miRNAs (miR-31, miR-125b, miR-200 and miR-205) which downregulate oncogenic proteins. Cancer-initiating cells (CSCs) were first isolated from breast cancer tumors and are considered the seed-cells of tumor development [31]. While CSCs are similar to normal somatic stem cells in that they are capable of asymmetric cell division and the efflux of small molecules, they have more phenotypic plasticity. The family of miRNAs known as let-7 was demonstrated to be a master regulator of self-renewal and tumor-seeding ability [32]. Likewise, the process of epithelial to mesenchymal transition (EMT) which enables tumorigenicity and invasion, was facilitated via transforming growth factor β2 (TGF-β2) and Zeb1 transcription factor mediated repression of the miR-200 and miR-141; two miRNAs which are responsible for epithelial differentiation [33].

In summary, reflecting the cancer cells aim of aberrant, dysregulated gene expression needed for tumor cell survival and proliferation, a global downregulation of all miRNAs is observed in cancer. In tumor cells, the main mechanism by which global miRNA production is suppressed is via the upregulation of miRNAs that target the crucial miRNA biogenesis enzyme Dicer, miR-103 and miR-107 [34]. Likewise, chromatin remodeling that results in an increase in miRNAs that support EMT and self-renewal rather than continuation of a differentiated cell type is observed [35].

5. miRNAs affecting breast cancer chemotherapy efficacy and resistance

Chemoresistance is the primary cause of treatment failure in breast cancer. Dysregulation of some miRNAs can result in increases in drug efflux, alter drug targets and energy metabolism, stimulate DNA repair pathways and evasion of apoptosis and result in loss of cell cycle control. The first BC drug was a DNA-replication blocker called doxorubicin. Resistance to doxorubicin correlated with downregulation of miR-505, miR-128, and miR-145 tumor suppressors [36–41]. In contrast, miR-663, miR-181a, and miR-106b are oncogenic miRNAs whose downregulation resulted in enhancement of doxorubicin sensitivity in formerly resistant cells [41–43]. Like doxorubicin, cisplatin inhibits DNA replication and was also one of the first established therapies for BC. Upregulation of miR-345 and miR-7 contribute to cisplatin-resistance, while miR-302b can sensitize resistant cells to cisplatin therapy [44, 45]. A list of miRNA expression levels and targets of BC drug resistant is listed in **Table 1**.

In addition to doxorubicin and cisplatin, efficacy of the chemotherapeutic agents docetaxel and paclitaxel which inhibit microtubule formation during cell division, can also be compromised by miRNAs. Downregulation of miR-34a, miR-100, and miR-30c were observed in paclitaxel-resistant BC cell while the upregulation of miR-129-3p was found to contribute to resistance [57–61].

In ER+ breast cancer, *de novo* and acquired resistance to conventional endocrine therapies such as aromatase inhibitors, fulvestrant and tamoxifen, can occur in more than 30% of patients [63]. Evidence suggests that resistance to these drugs is in part mediated by miRNAs. As most BC patients have high estrogen receptor-α (ER-α) expression, targeting ER-α signaling is a critical therapy. Resistance to tamoxifen, an agent which blocks interaction between estrogen and estrogen receptor is associated with the downregulation of the following tumor suppressor miRNAs: miR-15a, miR-16, miR-214, miR-320, miR-342, miR-451, miR-873,

miRNA	BC therapy	Targets	Level	Mechanism/Refs.
miR-200	Carboplatin	Zeb	↓	Reverses EMT [46]
miR-345	Cisplatin	MRP1	↓	Not yet characterized [45]
miR-7				
miR-302b	Cisplatin	E2F1 (direct)	↓	Inhibit cell cycle progression [44]
		ATM (indirect)		
miR-24	Cisplatin	BimL F1H1	↑	Promotes EMT and cancer stem cells [47]
miR-106b~25 cluster	Doxorubicin	EP300	↑	Activates EMT [43]
miR-128	Doxorubicin	Bmi-1 ABCC5	↓	Increases apoptosis [48]
miR-145	Doxorubicin	MRP1	↓	Induces intracellular doxorubicin accumulation [36]
miR-181a	Doxorubicin	Bcl-2	↓	Increases apoptosis [41]
miR-181a	Doxorubicin	Bax	↑	Inhibits apoptosis [49]
miR-25	Doxorubicin	ULK1	↑	Inhibits autophagy [50]
miR-326	Doxorubicin	MDR-1	↓	Downregulates MRP-1 [51]
miR-505	Doxorubicin	Akt3 (indirect)	↓	Not yet investigated [37]
miR-644a	Doxorubicin	CTBP1	↓	Inhibits EMT [52]
miR-663	Doxorubicin	HSPG2	↑	Inhibits apoptosis [42]
miR-129-3p	Docetaxel	CP100	↑	Reduces cell cycle arrest and apoptosis [53]
miR-34a	Docetaxel	BCL-2 CCND1	↑	Inhibit apoptosis [54]
miR-484	Gemcitabine	CDA	↓	Promote proliferation and cell-cycle redistribution [55]
miR-218	MDR	Survivin	↓	Enhance apoptosis [56]
miR-100	Paclitaxel	mTOR	↓	Enhance cell cycle arrest and apoptosis [57]
miR-125b	Paclitaxel	Sema4C	↓	Reverses EMT [58]
miR-125b	Taxol	Bak1	↑	Inhibits apoptosis [59]
miR-30c	Doxorubicin	TWF1 (PTK9) VIM IL-11	↓	Reverses EMT [60]
	Paclitaxel			
miR-34a	Doxorubicin	HDAC1HDAC7	↑	Inhibits autophagic cell death [61]
	Cisplatin			

Abbreviations: Expression level of miRs: upregulation (↑) or downregulation (↓) of miRNAs in breast cancer therapy. The reference of each miR is included in the table. Table adapted from Hu et al. [62].

Table 1.
miRNAs involved in the regulation of common breast cancer drugs.

miRNA-375, miR-378a-3p, and miR-574-3p [64–71] .In contrast, oncogenic miRs: miR-101, miR-221/222, miR-301, and miRNAs-C19MC were highly expressed in tamoxifen resistant cells [72–75]. In addition, both the humanized monoclonal antibody targeting HER2 named trastuzumab, as well as lapatinib, which is a small-molecule tyrosine kinase inhibitor targeting both HER2 and epithelial growth factor receptor (EGFR), improve therapeutic outcome but result in resistance after 1 year.

Resistance to these two drugs is correlated with an upregulation of miR-21, miR-221 and miR-375 [76–80].

The role of miRNA in chemotherapeutic resistance is associated with the modification of drug transporters which has a net effect of drug efflux out of the cell via exosomes as well as modifications of autophagy and apoptosis pathways which lead to enhanced survival, the promotion of growth factors and activation EMT [81]. The tumor microenvironment which consists of the surrounding stromal cells serve as the normal foundation upon which the deviant tumor "house" is constructed supplying it with blood vessels, signaling molecules and ECM. Exosomes transport bioactive molecules and mediate cellular communication in the tumor microenvironment, facilitating a more cancerous and recalcitrant milieu [82]. For example, exosome-derived miRNAs such as miR-222 transfer doxorubicin-resistance by inhibiting PTEN in recipient cells, 22 miRNAs were concentrated in exosomes and correlated to chemotherapy resistance [83]. While the major function of exosomes in the context of BC and drug resistance is the shuttling of drugs out of the tumor, exosomes can also be bio-hacked for use as a prime chemotherapy delivery system [84–86].

In summary, in the context of breast cancer, tumor cells regulate miRNAs in a way that promotes tumor survival, growth and invasion. Aside from a global down-regulation of most miRNAs and especially tumor suppressor miRNAs, oncogenic miRNAs are increased and often exported via exosomes where they are taken up by non-cancerous cells, transforming the local environment to a pro-cancer milieu. Knowing how BC cells regulate miRNAs opens the door for potential therapies that target oncogenic miRNAs (antagomirs) or add back tumor suppresser miRNAs (mimic miRNAs). The targeting of miRs in breast cancer is discussed in the following section.

6. miRNAs as breast cancer therapy

As reviewed in this chapter, miRNAs are dynamically regulated in BC and can also contribute to drug resistance. Therefore, interventions that disrupt activities of dysregulated miRNAs offer promising targets for novel therapeutics in the form of mimics or antagomirs. In addition, mature miRNAs and their precursors can also be targeted by small molecules. In general, there are two strategies for targeting miRNA in BC. In the first strategy, tumor suppressor miRNAs which are down regulated by tumor cells can be added back to the tumor microenvironment using chemically synthesized miRNA mimics which imitate endogenous mature double-stranded miRNA [87]. MiRNA mimics could be delivered in viral vectors which would allow extended expression. The second strategy is to target oncogenic miRNAs which are highly expressed and exported by tumor cells. In this strategy, oligonucleotides, locked-nucleic-acids antisense oligonucleotides (LNAs), miRNA sponges, multiple-target anti-miRNA antisense oligo-deoxyribonucleotides (MTg-AMOs), miRNA-masking and nanoparticles are used to target for degradation or impede aberrantly expressed oncogenic miRNAs from reaching their targets [88–91].

As previously mentioned, the majority of highly expressed, dysregulated miRNAs in tumor cells are oncomirs, or those that support tumorigenesis, while tumor suppressor miRNAs are suppressed [92]. For example, miR-155 is an oncogenic miRNA upregulated in BC tumor tissue. Targeting of miR-155 with an antisense oligonucleotide (miR-155) in a BC cell line blocked proliferation and augmented apoptosis [93]. MiR-892b is an example of a tumor suppressor miRNA that is significantly downregulated in BC tissue specimens. By supplementing miR-892b "mimics" in BC cells, a decrease in tumor growth, metastases rate, and angiogenesis was observed. MiR-892b mimic blocked impeded tumorigenesis by attenuating nuclear transcription factor kappa B (NF-kB) signaling [94]. Artificial miRNAs can also be constructed to inhibit targets that are not normally targeted by endogenous miRNAs. For example, a novel artificial miRNA (amiRNA) called miR-p-27-5p, which targets the 3′-UTR of cyclin-dependent kinase 4 (CDK4) mRNA, inhibited cell cycle progression via downregulation of CDK4 expression and suppression of retinoblastoma protein (RB1) phosphorylation [95]. Likewise, an a miRNA against a C-X-C motif chemokine receptor 4 (CXCR4) inserted into an expression vector reduced CXCR4 expression and suppressed migration and invasion of BC cells [96]. While in vitro experiments provide proof of concept for further development of miRNA targeting in oncogenic diseases, only clinical trial results can determine whether miRNA therapy is truly efficacious. Patents, clinical trials and biopharmaceutical companies invested in the development of miRNA therapies are summarized by Chakraborty *et al*, [97]. A seminal trial for miRNA replacement therapy took place employing the tumor suppressor miR-34 mimic (MRX34). MRX34 was formulated for intravenous injection using a liposome delivery system for patients with metastatic liver cancer. MRX34 along with dexamethasone was associated with safety and showed evidence of antitumor activity in a subset of patients with refractory advanced solid tumors [98]. However, there were adverse events in the trial which indicate the need for alternative approaches in formulation design and delivery.

In summary, there is much research to be done in the emerging field of miRNA therapeutics. Drug developers, pharmacists, physicians and molecular biologists must work together to develop novel strategies for miRNA delivery that is more targeted and controlled in order to mitigate off-target effects by affecting only cell signaling of targeted tumor cells.

7. miRNAs as breast cancer biomarkers

MiRNAs that maintain a stable presence in the serum are referred to as "circulating" miRNAs. Thus, in addition to therapeutic targeting, many studies have reported utility of miRNAs in the context of BC as biomarkers for diagnostic, prognostic, or predictive of drug efficacy. In this final section, miRNAs currently being used as biomarkers in the context of BC are discussed.

In the context of diagnostics, the current gold standard for BC is mammography. However, many women avoid mammograms for fear of pain or inconvenience in scheduling thus rendering assays performed on less invasive, routine blood draws amenable to early screening for BC. Global profiling of circulating miRNAs in early-stage ER+ BC (n = 48) and age-matched healthy controls (n = 24) revealed a panel of nine miRNAs (miR-15a, miR-18a, miR-107, miR-133a, miR-139-5p, miR-143, miR-145, miR-365 and miR-425) that discriminated between patients with early-stage ER+ BC and healthy controls [99]. A study in Japan performed on serum (n = 1280 BC, n = 2836 non-cancer controls) found a combination of five miRNAs: miR-1246, miR-1307-3p, miR-4634, miR-6861-5p and miR-6875-5p, could predict breast cancer with a sensitivity of 97.3% overall, 98% sensitivity for early stage BC and a specificity of 82.9% and accuracy of 89.7% [100]. A study based in Prague (n = 63 early stage BC, n = 21 non cancer controls) found that several oncogenic miRNAs were significantly elevated in early stage BC; including: miR-155, miR-19a, miR-181b, and miR-24 and unsurprisingly, their expression dropped following surgical resection of the tumor [101]. A study in Singapore performed global profiling

Source	miRNA	Expression/Refs	DX	PX	PR	VA
Blood	miR-195, let-7 and -155	↑ in BC [108]	Y	N	N	N
Serum	miR-214	Indicates malignant from benign and healthy [109]	Y	N	N	N
Plasma	miR-127-3p, -376a, -148b, -409-3p, -652 and -801	↑ in BC [110]	Y	N	N	Y
Plasma	miR-148b, -133a, and -409-3p	↑ in BC [111]	Y	N	N	Y
Serum	miR-15a	↑ in BC [99]	Y	N	N	Y
	miR-18a, -107, -425, -133a, -139-5p, -143, -145, and -365	↓ in BC [99]				
Serum	miR-484	↑ in BC [112]	Y	N	N	Y
Serum	miR-1246, -1307-3p, and -6861-5p	↑ in BC [100]	Y	N	N	Y
	miR-4634 and -6875-5p	↓ in BC [100]				
Serum	miR-155, -19a, -181b, and -24	↑ in BC [101]	Y	N	N	N
Serum	miR-1, -92a, -133a, and -133b	↑ in BC [102]	Y	N	N	Y
Plasma	miR-505-5p, -125b-5p, -21-5p, and -96-5p	↑ in BC [113]	Y	N	N	Y
Serum	let-7c	↓ in BC [103]	Y	N	N	N
Serum	miR-182	↑ in BC [114]	Y	N	N	N
Blood	miR-138	↑ in BC [115]	Y	N	N	N
Serum	miR-155	Correlates w/PR status [116]	Y	N	N	N
Serum	miR-21, -126, -155, -199a, and -335	Associated w/ histological tumor grade and sex hormone receptor expression [117]	Y	N	N	N
Serum; Plasma	miR-4270, -1225-5p, -188-5p, -1202, -4281, -1207-5p, -642b-3p, -1290, and -3141	↑ in BC and correlates w/stage and molecular subtype [118]	Y	N	N	Y
Serum	miR-202 and let-7b	↑ expression in BC and correlates w/ tumor aggressive and overall survival [119]	Y	Y	N	N
Serum	miR-148b-3p and -652-3p	↓ in the BC [120]	Y	Y	N	Y
	miR-10b-5p	↑ levels correlate w/ poor prognosis [120]				
Serum	miR-18b, -103, -107, and -652	Associated w/tumor relapse and overall survival in TNBC [105]	Y	Y	N	Y
Plasma	miR-10b and -373	↑ in breast cancer w/ LN metastasis [121]	Y	Y	N	Y
Serum	miR-10b, 34a, and -155	Correlates w/ tumor stage and/or metastasis [122]	Y	Y	N	N

Source	miRNA	Expression/Refs	DX	PX	PR	VA
Serum	miR-29b-2, miR-155, miR -197 and miR -205	Correlates w/tumor grade and metastasis [123]	Y	Y	N	N
Serum	miR-92a	↓ in BC, LN metastasis [124]	Y	Y	N	N
	miR-21	↑ in BC, LN metastasis [124]				
Serum	miR-21-5p, -375, -205-5p, and -194-5p	↑ in recurrent BC [125]	Y	Y	N	Y
	miR-382-5p, -376c-3p, and -411-5p	↓ in recurrent BC [125]				
Serum	miR-34a, -93, -373, -17, and -155	Expression correlated w/metastasis and HER2, PR, and ER status [126]	Y	N	N	N
Serum	miR-125b	↑ expression in non-responsive [127]	Y	N	Y	N
Serum	miR-122	↓ in NR and pCR [128]	N	N	Y	Y
	miR-375	↑ in NR and pCR [128]				
Serum	miR-155	↑ in BC; ↓ post chemo [107]	Y	N	Y	N

Abbreviations: DX, diagnostic; PX, prognostic; PR, predictive; VA, validated; BC, breast cancer; ddPCR, droplet digital PCR; DS, deep sequencing; ER, estrogen receptor; HER2, human epidermal growth factor receptor 2; LN, lymph node; miRNA (miR), microRNA; PR, progesterone receptor; qRT-PCR, quantitative reverse transcriptase real-time PCR; TNBC, triple-negative breast cancer; NR, non-relapse; pCR, Pathologic complete response.

Table 2.
Circulating miRNAs; diagnostic, prognostic, predictive and validated biomarkers in breast cancer.

of miRNA expression in BC tumor tissue, non-tumor tissue and serum samples obtained from BC patients (n = 132) and from healthy controls (n = 123) revealed miR-1, miR-92a, miR-133a and miR-133b as significantly upregulated diagnostic markers in BC sera [102]. In addition to upregulation of oncogenic miRNAs, tumor suppressor Let-7c was decreased in BC tissue and sera according to a study performed in China (n = 90 BC, n = 64 controls) [103]. Although some studies have suggested that let-7 and miR-195 restoration may be therapeutic, results of Qattan et al. in 2017 [104] supported literature indicating that tumor cells export hsa-miR-195 and let-7 miRNAs. While the data of this study did not generally support the use of these miRNAs as therapies, it suggested that these markers may be the most robust markers to use in a blood-based screen for the early detection of TNBC and luminal breast cancer [104].

The definition of a prognostic biomarker is one that indicates recurrence or progression; such as chance of survival, independent of the course of therapy. In a study based in Germany, pre-operative serum (n = 102) and post-operative serum (n = 34) of BC patients was compared to healthy women (n = 37) or those with benign breast disease (n = 26). The mean follow-up time of for BC patients was 6.2 years. In this study, high expression of miR-202 positively correlated with reduced overall survival (poor prognosis). In a European study, genome-wide miRNA expression profiling using serum from TNBC patients (n = 130) and healthy controls (n = 30), revealed a four-miRNA signature (miR-18b, miR-103, miR-107 and miR-652) that predicted tumor recurrence and overall survival [105]. While few studies have investigated the use of miRNA serum expression levels as a predictive metric for treatment response, clinically relevant outcomes were revealed in the studies performed indicating the need for incentivizing investigations into miRNA biomarkers. For example, elevated miR-125b expression predicts poor prognosis, is associated with tumor size and TNM stage in HER2+ BC as well as poor responsiveness to paclitaxel-based neoadjuvant chemotherapy [106]. Therefore, miR-125b may be a potential predictor of clinical outcome, particularly in HER2+ BC patients receiving paclitaxel-based neoadjuvant chemotherapy. In another example, miR-155 was significantly increased in BC patients (n = 103) compared with healthy normal (n = 55). Post-surgical resection and four cycles of chemotherapy, a subset of BC patient sera (n = 29) were collected to evaluate the effects of clinical treatment on serum levels of candidate miRNAs. Decreased levels of circulating miR-155 post-treatment was associated with response to therapy and stable disease [107].

In summary, the data from these studies and others suggest that BC patients with novel miRNA signatures correlating with poor prognosis are not receiving adequate treatment and should be selected for inclusion in novel randomized clinical trials for the chance to receive alternative life-saving therapies. **Table 2** summarizes studies revealing statistically significant regulation of circulating miRNAs with diagnostic (DX), prognostic (PX), predictive biomarkers (PR) potential for BC. Some studies were validated (VA) with alternative cohorts.

8. Conclusions

In conclusion, this chapter provided an overview of the most recent studies describing the dynamic roles of miRNAs in the context of BC. This overview demonstrates that just as miRNAs are integral to maintaining normal homeostasis, they are simultaneously sensitive to changes in overall physiology and local micro-environments thus studying them will likely lead to insight into the unique manifestation of BC in an individual. Given that they are actively released by tumor cells into the circulatory system, both monitoring and targeting miRNAs enables the diagnosis and monitoring of BC as well as the opportunity for the development of novel therapeutics. Future studies should employ well standardized methods for sample collection and multi-center global miRNA profiling to reveal novel nuances and robust results regarding miRNA signaling in the context of BC. Taken together, the emerging field of precision oncology may rely on understanding miRNA profiles.

Author details

Amal Qattan[1,2]

1 Department of Molecular Oncology, King Faisal Specialist Hospital and Research Centre, Riyadh, Saudi Arabia

2 Department of Biochemistry and Molecular Medicine, School of Medicine and Health Science (SMHS), GW University, Washington, DC, USA

*Address all correspondence to: aqattan5@gwu.edu; akattan@kfshrc.edu.sa

References

[1] Lee RC, Feinbaum RL, Ambros V. The *C. elegans* heterochronic gene lin-4 encodes small RNAs with antisense complementarity to lin-14. Cell. 1993;**75**:843-854

[2] Barbato S, Solaini G, Fabbri M. MicroRNAs in oncogenesis and tumor suppression. In: International Review of Cell and Molecular Biology. Galluzzi L, Vitale I, editors. MiRNAs in Differentiation and Development. Elsevier. 2017;**333**:229-268. DOI: 10.1016/bs.ircmb.2017.05.001. ISBN: 978-0-12-811870-2

[3] Kawahara Y. Human diseases caused by germline and somatic abnormalities in microRNA and microRNA-related genes. Congenital Anomalies (Kyoto). 2014;**54**:12-21. DOI: 10.1111/cga.12043

[4] Schmidt MF. Drug target miRNAs: Chances and challenges. Trends in Biotechnology. 2014;**32**:578-585. DOI: 10.1016/j.tibtech.2014.09.002

[5] WHO. Breast cancer. 2018. Available from: https://www.who.int/cancer/prevention/diagnosis-screening/breast-cancer/en/

[6] Moran Y, Agron M, Praher D, Technau U. The evolutionary origin of plant and animal microRNAs. Nature Ecology and Evolution. 2017;**1**:0027. DOI: 10.1038/s41559-016-0027

[7] Alvarez-Garcia I, Miska EA. MicroRNA functions in animal development and human disease. Development. 2005;**132**:4653-4662. DOI: 10.1242/dev.02073

[8] Lin Y, Zeng Y, Zhang F, Xue L, Huang Z, Li W, et al. Characterization of microRNA expression profiles and the discovery of novel microRNAs involved in cancer during human embryonic development. PLoS One. 2013;**8**:1-11. DOI: 10.1371/JOURNAL.PONE.0069230

[9] Rodriguez A, Griffiths-Jones S, Ashurst JL, Bradley A. Identification of mammalian microRNA host genes and transcription units. Genome Research. 2004;**14**:1902-1910. DOI: 10.1101/gr.2722704

[10] Hinske LC, França GS, Torres HAM, Ohara DT, Lopes-Ramos CM, Heyn J, et al. miRIAD—Integrating microRNA inter- and intragenic data. Database. 2014;**2014**:1-9. DOI: 10.1093/database/bau099

[11] Ha M, Kim VN. Regulation of microRNA biogenesis. Nature Reviews. Molecular Cell Biology. 2014;**15**:509-524. DOI: 10.1038/nrm3838

[12] Vasudevan S, Tong Y, Steitz JA. Switching from repression to activation: MicroRNAs can up-regulate translation. Science (80-). 2007;**318**:1931-1934. DOI: 10.1126/science.1149460

[13] Rüegger S, Großhans H. MicroRNA turnover: When, how, and why. Trends in Biochemical Sciences. 2012;**37**:436-446. DOI: 10.1016/j.tibs.2012.07.002

[14] Tsang J, Zhu J, van Oudenaarden A. MicroRNA-mediated feedback and feedforward loops are recurrent network motifs in mammals. Molecular Cell. 2007;**26**:753-767. DOI: 10.1016/j.molcel.2007.05.018

[15] Gulyaeva LF, Kushlinskiy NE. Regulatory mechanisms of microRNA expression. Journal of Translational Medicine. 2016;**14**:143. DOI: 10.1186/s12967-016-0893-x

[16] Goldberg AD, Allis CD, Bernstein E. Epigenetics: A landscape takes shape. Cell. 2007;**128**:635-638. DOI: 10.1016/j.cell.2007.02.006

[17] Messerschmidt DM, Knowles BB, Solter D. DNA methylation dynamics

during epigenetic reprogramming in the germline and preimplantation embryos. Genes & Development. 2014;**28**:812-828. DOI: 10.1101/gad.234294.113

[18] Weber B, Stresemann C, Brueckner B, Lyko F. Methylation of human microRNA genes in normal and neoplastic cells. Cell Cycle. 2007;**6**:1001-1005. DOI: 10.4161/cc.6.9.4209

[19] Morales S, Monzo M, Navarro A. Short conceptual overview epigenetic regulation mechanisms of microRNA expression. Biomolecular Concepts. 2017;**8**:203-212. DOI: 10.1515/bmc-2017-0024

[20] Wilk G, Braun R. regQTLs: Single nucleotide polymorphisms that modulate microRNA regulation of gene expression in tumors. PLoS Genetics. 2018;**14**:e1007837. DOI: 10.1371/journal.pgen.1007837

[21] CHEN T. The role of MicroRNA in chemical carcinogenesis. Journal of Environmental Science and Health, Part C. 2010;**28**:89-124. DOI: 10.1080/10590501.2010.481477

[22] Hansen KF, Sakamoto K, Obrietan K. MicroRNAs: A potential interface between the circadian clock and human health. Genome Medicine. 2011;**3**:10. DOI: 10.1186/gm224

[23] Cruz-Roa A, Gilmore H, Basavanhally A, Feldman M, Ganesan S, Shih NNC, et al. Accurate and reproducible invasive breast cancer detection in whole-slide images: A deep learning approach for quantifying tumor extent. Scientific Reports. 2017;**7**:46450. DOI: 10.1038/srep46450

[24] Russnes HG, Lingjærde OC, Børresen-Dale A-L, Caldas C. Breast cancer molecular stratification. The American Journal of Pathology. 2017;**187**:2152-2162. DOI: 10.1016/j.ajpath.2017.04.022

[25] Jemal A, Bray F, Center MM, Ferlay J, Ward E, Forman D. Global cancer statistics. CA: A Cancer Journal for Clinicians. 2011;**61**:69-90. DOI: 10.3322/caac.20107

[26] Tahiri A, Leivonen S-K, Lüders T, Steinfeld I, Ragle Aure M, Geisler J, et al. Deregulation of cancer-related miRNAs is a common event in both benign and malignant human breast tumors. Carcinogenesis. 2014;**35**:76-85. DOI: 10.1093/carcin/bgt333

[27] Coates AS, Winer EP, Goldhirsch A, Gelber RD, Gnant M, Piccart-Gebhart M, et al. Panel members: Tailoring therapies—Improving the management of early breast cancer: St Gallen international expert consensus on the primary therapy of early breast cancer 2015. Annals of Oncology. 2015;**26**:1533-1546. DOI: 10.1093/annonc/mdv221

[28] Howard EW, Yang X. microRNA regulation in estrogen receptor-positive breast cancer and endocrine therapy. Biological Procedures Onlin. 2018;**20**:17. DOI: 10.1186/s12575-018-0082-9

[29] Hemmatzadeh M, Mohammadi H, Jadidi-Niaragh F, Asghari F, Yousefi M. The role of oncomirs in the pathogenesis and treatment of breast cancer. Biomedicine & Pharmacotherapy. 2016;**78**:129-139. DOI: 10.1016/j.biopha.2016.01.026

[30] Wang W, Luo Y. MicroRNAs in breast cancer: Oncogene and tumor suppressors with clinical potential. Journal of Zhejiang University. Science. B. 2015;**16**:18-31. DOI: 10.1631/jzus.B1400184

[31] Al-Hajj M, Wicha MS, Benito-Hernandez A, Morrison SJ, Clarke MF. Prospective identification of tumorigenic breast cancer cells. Proceedings of the National Academy of Sciences. 2003;**100**:3983-3988. DOI: 10.1073/pnas.0530291100

[32] Yu F, Yao H, Zhu P, Zhang X, Pan Q, Gong C, et al. Let-7 regulates self renewal and tumorigenicity of breast cancer cells. Cell. 2007;**131**:1109-1123. DOI: 10.1016/J.CELL.2007.10.054

[33] Burk U, Schubert J, Wellner U, Schmalhofer O, Vincan E, Spaderna S, et al. A reciprocal repression between ZEB1 and members of the miR-200 family promotes EMT and invasion in cancer cells. EMBO Reports. 2008;**9**:582-589. DOI: 10.1038/embor.2008.74

[34] Martello G, Rosato A, Ferrari F, Manfrin A, Cordenonsi M, Dupont S, et al. A microRNA targeting dicer for metastasis control. Cell. 2010;**141**:1195-1207. DOI: 10.1016/j.cell.2010.05.017

[35] Song SJ, Poliseno L, Song MS, Ala U, Webster K, Ng C, et al. MicroRNA-antagonism regulates breast cancer stemness and metastasis via TET-family-dependent chromatin remodeling. Cell. 2013;**154**:311-324. DOI: 10.1016/j.cell.2013.06.026

[36] Gao M, Miao L, Liu M, Li C, Yu C, Yan H, et al. miR-145 sensitizes breast cancer to doxorubicin by targeting multidrug resistance-associated protein-1. Oncotarget. 2016;7:59714-59726. DOI: 10.18632/oncotarget.10845

[37] Yamamoto Y, Yoshioka Y, Minoura K, Takahashi R, Takeshita F, Taya T, et al. An integrative genomic analysis revealed the relevance of microRNA and gene expression for drug-resistance in human breast cancer cells. Molecular Cancer. 2011;**10**:135. DOI: 10.1186/1476-4598-10-135

[38] Vivanco I, Sawyers CL. The phosphatidylinositol 3-kinase–AKT pathway in human cancer. Nature Reviews. Cancer. 2002;**2**:489-501. DOI: 10.1038/nrc839

[39] Yuan X-J, Whang YE. PTEN sensitizes prostate cancer cells to death receptor-mediated and drug-induced apoptosis through a FADD-dependent pathway. Oncogene. 2002;**21**:319-327. DOI: 10.1038/sj.onc.1205054

[40] Wan X, Yokoyama Y, Shinohara A, Takahashi Y, Tamaya T. PTEN augments staurosporine-induced apoptosis in PTEN-null Ishikawa cells by downregulating PI3K/Akt signaling pathway. Cell Death and Differentiation. 2002;**9**:414-420. DOI: 10.1038/sj/cdd/4400982

[41] Zhu Y, Wu J, Li S, Ma R, Cao H, Ji M, et al. The function role of miR-181a in Chemosensitivity to Adriamycin by targeting Bcl-2 in low-invasive breast cancer cells. Cellular Physiology and Biochemistry. 2013;**32**:1225-1237. DOI: 10.1159/000354521

[42] Hu H, Li S, Cui X, Lv X, Jiao Y, Yu F, et al. The overexpression of hypomethylated miR-663 induces chemotherapy resistance in human breast cancer cells by targeting heparin sulfate proteoglycan 2 (HSPG2). The Journal of Biological Chemistry. 2013;**288**:10973-10985. DOI: 10.1074/jbc.M112.434340

[43] Zhou Y, Hu Y, Yang M, Jat P, Li K, Lombardo Y, et al. The miR-106b~25 cluster promotes bypass of doxorubicin-induced senescence and increase in motility and invasion by targeting the E-cadherin transcriptional activator EP300. Cell Death and Differentiation. 2014;**21**:462-474. DOI: 10.1038/cdd.2013.167

[44] Cataldo A, Cheung DG, Balsari A, Tagliabue E, Coppola V, Iorio MV, et al. miR-302b enhances breast cancer cell sensitivity to cisplatin by regulating E2F1 and the cellular DNA damage response. Oncotarget. 2016;**7**:786-797. DOI: 10.18632/oncotarget.6381

[45] Pogribny IP, Filkowski JN, Tryndyak VP, Golubov A, Shpyleva SI, Kovalchuk O. Alterations of microRNAs and their

targets are associated with acquired resistance of MCF-7 breast cancer cells to cisplatin. International Journal of Cancer. 2010;**127**:1785-1794. DOI: 10.1002/ijc.25191

[46] Nurse P. Cyclin dependent kinases and cell cycle control (Nobel Lecture) Copyright © The Nobel Foundation, 2002. We thank the Nobel foundation, Stockholm, for permission to print this lecture. Chembiochem. 2002;**3**:596. DOI: 10.1002/1439-7633(20020703)3:7<596::AID-CBIC596>3.0.CO;2-U

[47] Bai W-D, Ye X-M, Zhang M-Y, Zhu H-Y, Xi W-J, Huang X, et al. MiR-200c suppresses TGF-β signaling and counteracts trastuzumab resistance and metastasis by targeting ZNF217 and ZEB1 in breast cancer. International Journal of Cancer. 2014;**135**:1356-1368. DOI: 10.1002/ijc.28782

[48] Zhu Y, Yu F, Jiao Y, Feng J, Tang W, Yao H, et al. Reduced miR-128 in breast tumor-initiating cells induces chemotherapeutic resistance via Bmi-1 and ABCC5. Clinical Cancer Research. 2011;**17**:7105-7115. DOI: 10.1158/1078-0432.CCR-11-0071

[49] Clarke R, Skaar TC, Bouker KB, Davis N, Lee YR, Welch JN, et al. Molecular and pharmacological aspects of antiestrogen resistance. The Journal of Steroid Biochemistry and Molecular Biology. 2001;**76**:71-84

[50] Wang Z, Wang N, Liu P, Chen Q, Situ H, Xie T, et al. MicroRNA-25 regulates chemoresistance-associated autophagy in breast cancer cells, a process modulated by the natural autophagy inducer isoliquiritigenin. Oncotarget. 2014;**5**:7013-7026. DOI: 10.18632/oncotarget.2192

[51] Liang Z, Wu H, Xia J, Li Y, Zhang Y, Huang K, et al. Involvement of miR-326 in chemotherapy resistance of breast cancer through modulating expression of multidrug resistance-associated protein 1. Biochemical Pharmacology. 2010;**79**:817-824. DOI: 10.1016/j.bcp.2009.10.017

[52] Reed JC. Bcl-2 family proteins. Oncogene. 1998;**17**:3225-3236. DOI: 10.1038/sj.onc.1202591

[53] Zhang Y, Wang Y, Wei Y, Li M, Yu S, Ye M, et al. MiR-129-3p promotes docetaxel resistance of breast cancer cells via CP110 inhibition. Scientific Reports. 2015;**5**:15424. DOI: 10.1038/srep15424

[54] Li L, Yuan L, Luo J, Gao J, Guo J, Xie X. MiR-34a inhibits proliferation and migration of breast cancer through down-regulation of Bcl-2 and SIRT1. Clinical and Experimental Medicine. 2013;**13**:109-117. DOI: 10.1007/s10238-012-0186-5

[55] Ye F-G, Song C-G, Cao Z-G, Xia C, Chen D-N, Chen L, et al. Cytidine deaminase axis modulated by miR-484 differentially regulates cell proliferation and Chemoresistance in breast cancer. Cancer Research. 2015;**75**:1504-1515. DOI: 10.1158/0008-5472.CAN-14-2341

[56] Hu Y, Xu K, Yagüe E. miR-218 targets survivin and regulates resistance to chemotherapeutics in breast cancer. Breast Cancer Research and Treatment. 2015;**151**:269-280. DOI: 10.1007/s10549-015-3372-9

[57] Zhang B, Zhao R, He Y, Fu X, Fu L, Zhu Z, et al. Micro RNA 100 sensitizes luminal a breast cancer cells to paclitaxel treatment in part by targeting mTOR. Oncotarget. 2016;**7**:5702-5714. DOI: 10.18632/oncotarget.6790

[58] Yang Q, Wang Y, Lu X, Zhao Z, Zhu L, Chen S, et al. MiR-125b regulates epithelial-mesenchymal transition via targeting Sema4C in paclitaxel-resistant breast cancer cells. Oncotarget. 2015;**6**:3268-3279. DOI: 10.18632/oncotarget.3065

[59] Zhou M, Liu Z, Zhao Y, Ding Y, Liu H, Xi Y, et al. MicroRNA-125b confers the resistance of breast cancer cells to paclitaxel through suppression of pro-apoptotic Bcl-2 antagonist killer 1 (Bak1) expression. The Journal of Biological Chemistry. 2010;**285**:21496-21507. DOI: 10.1074/jbc.M109.083337

[60] Bockhorn J, Dalton R, Nwachukwu C, Huang S, Prat A, Yee K, et al. MicroRNA-30c inhibits human breast tumour chemotherapy resistance by regulating TWF1 and IL-11. Nature Communications. 2013;**4**:1393. DOI: 10.1038/ncomms2393

[61] Wu M-Y, Fu J, Xiao X, Wu J, Wu R-C. MiR-34a regulates therapy resistance by targeting HDAC1 and HDAC7 in breast cancer. Cancer Letters. 2014;**354**:311-319. DOI: 10.1016/j.canlet.2014.08.031

[62] Hu W, Tan C, He Y, Zhang G, Xu Y, Tang J. Functional miRNAs in breast cancer drug resistance. OncoTargets and Therapy. 2018;**11**:1529-1541. DOI: 10.2147/OTT.S152462

[63] EBCTCG, Davies C, Godwin J, Gray R, Clarke M, Cutter D, et al. Relevance of breast cancer hormone receptors and other factors to the efficacy of adjuvant tamoxifen: patient-level meta-analysis of randomised trials. Lancet. 2011;**378**:771. DOI: 10.1016/S0140-6736(11)60993-8

[64] Cui J, Yang Y, Li H, Leng Y, Qian K, Huang Q, et al. MiR-873 regulates ERα transcriptional activity and tamoxifen resistance via targeting CDK3 in breast cancer cells. Oncogene. 2015;**34**:3895-3907. DOI: 10.1038/onc.2014.430

[65] Cittelly DM, Das PM, Salvo VA, Fonseca JP, Burow ME, Jones FE. Oncogenic HER2{Delta}16 suppresses miR-15a/16 and deregulates BCL-2 to promote endocrine resistance of breast tumors. Carcinogenesis. 2010;**31**:2049-2057. DOI: 10.1093/carcin/bgq192

[66] Lü M, Ding K, Zhang G, Yin M, Yao G, Tian H, et al. MicroRNA-320a sensitizes tamoxifen-resistant breast cancer cells to tamoxifen by targeting ARPP-19 and ERRγ. Scientific Reports. 2015;**5**:8735. DOI: 10.1038/srep08735

[67] Liu Z-R, Song Y, Wan L-H, Zhang Y-Y, Zhou L-M. Over-expression of miR-451a can enhance the sensitivity of breast cancer cells to tamoxifen by regulating 14-3-3ζ, estrogen receptor α, and autophagy. Life Sciences. 2016;**149**:104-113. DOI: 10.1016/j.lfs.2016.02.059

[68] Yu X, Luo A, Liu Y, Wang S, Li Y, Shi W, et al. MiR-214 increases the sensitivity of breast cancer cells to tamoxifen and fulvestrant through inhibition of autophagy. Molecular Cancer. 2015;**14**:208. DOI: 10.1186/s12943-015-0480-4

[69] Ward A, Balwierz A, Zhang JD, Küblbeck M, Pawitan Y, Hielscher T, et al. Re-expression of microRNA-375 reverses both tamoxifen resistance and accompanying EMT-like properties in breast cancer. Oncogene. 2013;**32**:1173-1182. DOI: 10.1038/onc.2012.128

[70] Ikeda K, Horie-Inoue K, Ueno T, Suzuki T, Sato W, Shigekawa T, et al. miR-378a-3p modulates tamoxifen sensitivity in breast cancer MCF-7 cells through targeting GOLT1A. Scientific Reports. 2015;**5**:13170. DOI: 10.1038/srep13170

[71] Ujihira T, Ikeda K, Suzuki T, Yamaga R, Sato W, Horie-Inoue K, et al. MicroRNA-574-3p, identified by microRNA library-based functional screening, modulates tamoxifen response in breast cancer. Scientific Reports. 2015;**5**:7641. DOI: 10.1038/srep07641

[72] Sachdeva M, Wu H, Ru P, Hwang L, Trieu V, Mo Y-Y. MicroRNA-101-mediated Akt activation and estrogen-independent growth. Oncogene. 2011;**30**:822-831. DOI: 10.1038/onc.2010.463

[73] Zugmaier G, Ennis BW, Deschauer B, Katz D, Knabbe C, Wilding G, et al. Transforming growth factors type β1 and β2 are equipotent growth inhibitors of human breast cancer cell lines. Journal of Cellular Physiology. 1989;**141**:353-361. DOI: 10.1002/jcp.1041410217

[74] McEarchern JA, Kobie JJ, Mack V, Wu RS, Meade-Tollin L, Arteaga CL, et al. Invasion and metastasis of a mammary tumor involves TGF-beta signaling. International Journal of Cancer. 2001;**91**:76-82

[75] Shi W, Gerster K, Alajez NM, Tsang J, Waldron L, Pintilie M, et al. MicroRNA-301 mediates proliferation and invasion in human breast Cancer. Cancer Research. 2011;**71**:2926-2937. DOI: 10.1158/0008-5472.CAN-10-3369

[76] Zhao Y, Liu H, Liu Z, Ding Y, Ledoux SP, Wilson GL, et al. Overcoming trastuzumab resistance in breast cancer by targeting dysregulated glucose metabolism. Cancer Research. 2011;**71**:4585-4597. DOI: 10.1158/0008-5472.CAN-11-0127

[77] Gong C, Yao Y, Wang Y, Liu B, Wu W, Chen J, et al. Up-regulation of *miR-21* mediates resistance to Trastuzumab therapy for breast cancer. The Journal of Biological Chemistry. 2011;**286**:19127-19137. DOI: 10.1074/jbc.M110.216887

[78] Dall P, Lenzen G, Gohler T, Lerchenmuller C, Feisel-Schwickardi G, Koch T, et al. Trastuzumab in the treatment of elderly patients with early breast cancer: Results from an observational study in Germany. Journal of Geriatric Oncology. 2015;**6**:462-469. DOI: 10.1016/j.jgo.2015.06.003

[79] De Mattos-Arruda L, Bottai G, Nuciforo PG, Di Tommaso L, Giovannetti E, Peg V, et al. MicroRNA-21 links epithelial-to-mesenchymal transition and inflammatory signals to confer resistance to neoadjuvant trastuzumab and chemotherapy in HER2-positive breast cancer patients. Oncotarget. 2015;**6**:37269-37280. DOI: 10.18632/oncotarget.5495

[80] Ye X-M, Zhu H-Y, Bai W-D, Wang T, Wang L, Chen Y, et al. Epigenetic silencing of miR-375 induces trastuzumab resistance in HER2-positive breast cancer by targeting IGF1R. BMC Cancer. 2014;**14**:134. DOI: 10.1186/1471-2407-14-134

[81] Russo F, Di Bella S, Nigita G, Macca V, Lagana A, Giugno R, et al. miRandola: extracellular circulating microRNAs database. PLoS One. 2012;7:e47786. DOI: 10.1371/journal.pone.0047786

[82] Falcone G, Felsani A, D'Agnano I. Signaling by exosomal microRNAs in cancer. Journal of Experimental and Clinical Cancer Research. 2015;**34**:32. DOI: 10.1186/s13046-015-0148-3

[83] Yu D, Wu Y, Zhang X, Lv M, Chen W, Chen X, et al. Exosomes from adriamycin-resistant breast cancer cells transmit drug resistance partly by delivering miR-222. Tumor Biology. 2016;**37**:3227-3235. DOI: 10.1007/s13277-015-4161-0

[84] Yang M, Chen J, Su F, Yu B, Su F, Lin L, et al. Microvesicles secreted by macrophages shuttle invasion-potentiating microRNAs into breast cancer cells. Molecular Cancer. 2011;**10**:117. DOI: 10.1186/1476-4598-10-117

[85] Federici C, Petrucci F, Caimi S, Cesolini A, Logozzi M, Borghi M, et al. Exosome release and low pH belong to a framework of resistance of human

melanoma cells to cisplatin. PLoS One. 2014;**9**:e88193. DOI: 10.1371/journal.pone.0088193

[86] Hannafon BN, Ding WQ. Intercellular communication by exosome-derived microRNAs in cancer. International Journal of Molecular Sciences. 2013;**14**:14240-14269. DOI: 10.3390/ijms140714240

[87] Bader AG, Brown D, Winkler M. The promise of microRNA replacement therapy. Cancer Research. 2010;**70**:7027-7030. DOI: 10.1158/0008-5472.CAN-10-2010

[88] Esau CC. Inhibition of microRNA with antisense oligonucleotides. Methods. 2008;**44**:55-60. DOI: 10.1016/j.ymeth.2007.11.001

[89] Elmén J, Lindow M, Schütz S, Lawrence M, Petri A, Obad S, et al. LNA-mediated microRNA silencing in non-human primates. Nature. 2008;**452**:896-899. DOI: 10.1038/nature06783

[90] Krützfeldt J, Rajewsky N, Braich R, Rajeev KG, Tuschl T, Manoharan M, et al. Silencing of microRNAs in vivo with 'antagomirs'. Nature. 2005;**438**:685-689. DOI: 10.1038/nature04303

[91] Majid S, Dahiya R. MicroRNA based therapeutic strategies for cancer: Emphasis on advances in renal cell carcinoma. In: MicroRNA Targeted Cancer Therapy. Cham: Springer International Publishing; 2014. pp. 175-188

[92] Romero-Cordoba S, Rodriguez-Cuevas S, Rebollar-Vega R, Quintanar-Jurado V, Maffuz-Aziz A, Jimenez-Sanchez G, et al. Identification and pathway analysis of microRNAs with No previous involvement in breast cancer. PLoS One. 2012;**7**:e31904. DOI: 10.1371/journal.pone.0031904

[93] Zheng S-R, Guo G-L, Zhai Q, Zou Z-Y, Zhang W. Effects of miR-155 antisense oligonucleotide on breast carcinoma cell line MDA-MB-157 and implanted tumors. Asian Pacific Journal of Cancer Prevention. 2013;**14**:2361-2366

[94] Jiang L, Yu L, Zhang X, Lei F, Wang L, Liu X, et al. miR-892b silencing activates NF-B and promotes aggressiveness in breast Cancer. Cancer Research. 2016;**76**:1101-1111. DOI: 10.1158/0008-5472.CAN-15-1770

[95] Tseng C-W, Huang H-C, Shih AC-C, Chang Y-Y, Hsu C-C, Chang J-Y, et al. Revealing the anti-tumor effect of artificial miRNA p-27-5p on human breast carcinoma cell line T-47D. International Journal of Molecular Sciences. 2012;**13**:6352-6369. DOI: 10.3390/ijms13056352

[96] Liang Z, Wu H, Reddy S, Zhu A, Wang S, Blevins D, et al. Blockade of invasion and metastasis of breast cancer cells via targeting CXCR4 with an artificial microRNA. Biochemical and Biophysical Research Communications. 2007;**363**:542-546. DOI: 10.1016/j.bbrc.2007.09.007

[97] Chakraborty C, Sharma AR, Sharma G, George C, Doss P, Lee S-S. Therapeutic miRNA and siRNA: Moving from bench to clinic as next generation medicine. 15 Sep 2017;**8**:132-143. DOI: 10.1016/j.omtn.2017.06.005

[98] Beg MS, Brenner AJ, Sachdev J, Borad M, Kang Y-K, Stoudemire J, et al. Phase I study of MRX34, a liposomal miR-34a mimic, administered twice weekly in patients with advanced solid tumors. Investigational New Drugs. 2017;**35**:180-188. DOI: 10.1007/s10637-016-0407-y

[99] Kodahl AR, Lyng MB, Binder H, Cold S, Gravgaard K, Knoop AS, et al. Novel circulating microRNA signature

as a potential non-invasive multi-marker test in ER-positive early-stage breast cancer: A case control study. Molecular Oncology. 2014;**8**:874-883. DOI: 10.1016/j.molonc.2014.03.002

[100] Shimomura A, Shiino S, Kawauchi J, Takizawa S, Sakamoto H, Matsuzaki J, et al. Novel combination of serum microRNA for detecting breast cancer in the early stage. Cancer Science. 2016;**107**:326-334. DOI: 10.1111/cas.12880

[101] Sochor M, Basova P, Pesta M, Dusilkova N, Bartos J, Burda P, et al. Oncogenic MicroRNAs: miR-155, miR-19a, miR-181b, and miR-24 enable monitoring of early breast cancer in serum. BMC Cancer. 2014;**14**:448. DOI: 10.1186/1471-2407-14-448

[102] Chan M, Liaw CS, Ji SM, Tan HH, Wong CY, Thike AA, et al. Identification of circulating MicroRNA signatures for breast cancer detection. Clinical Cancer Research. 2013;**19**:4477-4487. DOI: 10.1158/1078-0432.CCR-12-3401

[103] Li X-X, Gao S-Y, Wang P-Y, Zhou X, Li Y-J, Yu Y, et al. Reduced expression levels of let-7c in human breast cancer patients. Oncology Letters. 2015;**9**:1207-1212. DOI: 10.3892/ol.2015.2877

[104] Qattan A, Intabli H, Alkhayal W, Eltabache C, Tweigieri T, Amer SB. Robust expression of tumor suppressor miRNA's let-7 and miR-195 detected in plasma of Saudi female breast cancer patients. BMC Cancer. 2017;**17**:799. DOI: 10.1186/s12885-017-3776-5

[105] Kleivi Sahlberg K, Bottai G, Naume B, Burwinkel B, Calin GA, Borresen-Dale A-L, et al. A serum microRNA signature predicts tumor relapse and survival in triple-negative breast cancer patients. Clinical Cancer Research. 2015;**21**:1207-1214. DOI: 10.1158/1078-0432.CCR-14-2011

[106] Luo Y, Wang X, Niu W, Wang H, Wen Q, Fan S, et al. Elevated microRNA-125b levels predict a worse prognosis in HER2-positive breast cancer patients. Oncology Letters. 2017;**13**:867-874. DOI: 10.3892/ol.2016.5482

[107] Sun Y, Wang M, Lin G, Sun S, Li X, Qi J, et al. Serum MicroRNA-155 as a potential biomarker to track disease in breast cancer. PLoS One. 2012;**7**:e47003. DOI: 10.1371/journal.pone.0047003

[108] Heneghan HM, Miller N, Kelly R, Newell J, Kerin MJ. Systemic miRNA-195 differentiates breast cancer from other malignancies and is a potential biomarker for detecting noninvasive and early stage disease. The Oncologist. 2010;**15**:673-682. DOI: 10.1634/theoncologist.2010-0103

[109] Schwarzenbach H, Milde-Langosch K, Steinbach B, Müller V, Pantel K. Diagnostic potential of PTEN-targeting miR-214 in the blood of breast cancer patients. Breast Cancer Research and Treatment. 2012;**134**:933-941. DOI: 10.1007/s10549-012-1988-6

[110] Cuk K, Zucknick M, Madhavan D, Schott S, Golatta M, Heil J, et al. Plasma MicroRNA panel for minimally invasive detection of breast Cancer. PLoS One. 2013;**8**:e76729. DOI: 10.1371/journal.pone.0076729

[111] Shen J, Hu Q, Schrauder M, Yan L, Wang D, Liu S. Circulating miR-148b and miR-133a as biomarkers for breast cancer detection. Oncotarget. 2014;**5**:5284-5294. Available from: https://doi.org/10.18632/oncotarget.2014

[112] Zearo S, Kim E, Zhu Y, Zhao JT, Sidhu SB, Robinson BG, et al. MicroRNA-484 is more highly expressed in serum of early breast cancer patients compared to healthy volunteers. BMC Cancer. 2014;**14**:200. DOI: 10.1186/1471-2407-14-200

[113] Matamala N, Vargas MT, Gonzalez-Campora R, Minambres R, Arias JI, Menendez P, et al. Tumor microRNA expression profiling identifies circulating microRNAs for early breast cancer detection. Clinical Chemistry. 2015;**61**:1098-1106. DOI: 10.1373/clinchem.2015.238691

[114] Wang P-Y, Gong H-T, Li B-F, Lv C-L, Wang H-T, Zhou H-H, et al. Higher expression of circulating miR-182 as a novel biomarker for breast cancer. Oncology Letters. 2013;**6**:1681-1686. DOI: 10.3892/ol.2013.1593

[115] Waters PS, Dwyer RM, Brougham C, Glynn CL, Wall D, Hyland P, et al. Impact of tumour epithelial subtype on circulating microRNAs in breast cancer patients. PLoS One. 2014;**9**:e90605. DOI: 10.1371/journal.pone.0090605

[116] Zhu W, Qin W, Atasoy U, Sauter ER. Circulating microRNAs in breast cancer and healthy subjects. BMC Research Notes. 2009;**2**:89. DOI: 10.1186/1756-0500-2-89

[117] Wang F, Zheng Z, Guo J, Ding X. Correlation and quantitation of microRNA aberrant expression in tissues and sera from patients with breast tumor. Gynecologic Oncology. 2010;**119**:586-593. DOI: 10.1016/j.ygyno.2010.07.021

[118] Hamam R, Ali AM, Alsaleh KA, Kassem M, Alfayez M, Aldahmash A, et al. microRNA expression profiling on individual breast cancer patients identifies novel panel of circulating microRNA for early detection. Scientific Reports. 2016;**6**:25997. DOI: 10.1038/srep25997

[119] Joosse SA, Müller V, Steinbach B, Pantel K, Schwarzenbach H. Circulating cell-free cancer-testis MAGE-A RNA, BORIS RNA, let-7b and miR-202 in the blood of patients with breast cancer and benign breast diseases. British Journal of Cancer. 2014;**111**:909-917. DOI: 10.1038/bjc.2014.360

[120] Mangolini A, Ferracin M, Zanzi MV, Saccenti E, Ebnaof SO, Poma VV, et al. Diagnostic and prognostic microRNAs in the serum of breast cancer patients measured by droplet digital PCR. Biomarker Research. 2015;**3**:12. DOI: 10.1186/s40364-015-0037-0

[121] Chen W, Cai F, Zhang B, Barekati Z, Zhong XY. The level of circulating miRNA-10b and miRNA-373 in detecting lymph node metastasis of breast cancer: Potential biomarkers. Tumor Biology. 2013;**34**:455-462. DOI: 10.1007/s13277-012-0570-5

[122] Roth C, Rack B, Muller V, Janni W, Pantel K, Schwarzenbach H. Circulating microRNAs as blood-based markers for patients with primary and metastatic breast cancer. Breast Cancer Research. 2010;**12**:R90. DOI: 10.1186/bcr2766

[123] Shaker O, Maher M, Nassar Y, Morcos G, Gad Z. Role of microRNAs -29b-2, -155, -197 and -205 as diagnostic biomarkers in serum of breast cancer females. Gene. 2015;**560**:77-82. DOI: 10.1016/J.GENE.2015.01.062

[124] Si H, Sun X, Chen Y, Cao Y, Chen S, Wang H, et al. Circulating microRNA-92a and microRNA-21 as novel minimally invasive biomarkers for primary breast cancer. Journal of Cancer Research and Clinical Oncology. 2013;**139**:223-229. DOI: 10.1007/s00432-012-1315-y

[125] Huo D, Clayton W, Yoshimatsu T, Chen J, Olopade O. Identification of a circulating microRNA signature to distinguish recurrence in breast cancer patients. Oncotarget. 2016;7:55231-55248. https://doi.org/10.18632/oncotarget.10485

[126] Eichelser C, Flesch-Janys D, Chang-Claude J, Pantel K, Schwarzenbach H. Deregulated serum concentrations of circulating cell-free microRNAs miR-17, miR-34a, miR-155,

and miR-373 in human breast cancer development and progression. Clinical Chemistry. 2013;**59**:1489-1496. DOI: 10.1373/clinchem.2013.205161

[127] Wang H, Tan G, Dong L, Cheng L, Li K, Wang Z, et al. Circulating MiR-125b as a marker predicting chemoresistance in breast cancer. PLoS One. 2012;7:e34210. DOI: 10.1371/journal.pone.0034210

[128] Wu X, Somlo G, Yu Y, Palomares MR, Li A, Zhou W, et al. De novo sequencing of circulating miRNAs identifies novel markers predicting clinical outcome of locally advanced breast cancer. Journal of Translational Medicine. 2012;**10**:42. DOI: 10.1186/1479-5876-10-42

Section 3

Tumor Suppressor Proteins in Cell Signalling Pathways

Chapter 5

Regulation of HDACi–Triggered Autophagy by the Tumor Suppressor Protein p53

Maria Mrakovcic and Leopold F. Fröhlich

Abstract

Cancer is a complex genetic and epigenetic-based disease that has developed a multitude of mechanisms in evading cell death. Deregulation of apoptosis and autophagy are commonly encountered during the development of human tumors. Histone deacetylase inhibitors (HDACi) have been employed to reverse epigenetically deregulated gene expression caused by aberrant post-translational protein modifications. These interfere with histone acetyltransferase- and deacetylase-mediated acetylation of histone and non-histone proteins, and thereby exert a wide array of HDACi-stimulated cytotoxic effects. Key determinants of HDACi lethality that interfere with cellular growth in a multitude of tumor cells are apoptosis and autophagy. Currently, the factors that determine the mode of HDACi-elicited cell death are mostly unclear however. Experimental evidence of the last decade convincingly reports that the frequently mutated tumor suppressor protein p53 can act either as an activator or as an inhibitor of autophagy depending on its subcellular localization, and linked to its mode of action. Consistently, we recently described p53 as a regulatory switch that governs if histone deacetylase inhibitor-administered uterine sarcoma cells undergo autophagy or apoptosis. By highlighting this novel finding, we summarize in this chapter the role of p53-mediated signaling during the activation of the autophagic pathway in tumor cells in response to HDACi.

Keywords: p53, HDACi, autophagy, apoptosis, tumor

1. Introduction

Evading cell death has been defined as a cornerstone of cancer development [1, 2]. Exploring the pathogenetic mechanisms that determine different cell death modes therefore facilitated the avenue for increased specifically directed interference with these molecular pathways. Morphologically, apoptosis, autophagy, and necrosis could be distinguished as major categories of programmed cell death very early that either act mutually exclusive or in combination involving cross talk for the elimination of tumor cells. While apoptosis and necrosis lead to inevitable cellular demise, autophagy can have either a cytotoxic or a cytoprotective function [3]. Basal autophagy in normal eukaryotic cells provide a possibility to save energy and reuse damaged or aged macromolecules or organelles by redirecting them toward lysosomal degradation via so-called autophagosomes and can be triggered by nutrient-starving conditions [4, 5]. Thus, in early phases of tumorigenesis, autophagy obviously presumes a cytoprotective or pro-survival role by suppressing necrosis and inflammation with concomitant disruption of necrotic and apoptotic cell death induction [6, 7]. In later stages of irreversible tumor development however, autophagy may promote cell death by largely non-elucidated mechanisms that expedite the "self-degradation" program [8]. Disruption of autophagy in the latter case, which was recently enforced as novel strategy in chemotherapeutic cancer treatment, will advance the survival of tumor cells. This insight stresses the significance to confirm the context-reliant function of autophagy before initiating cancer therapy involving autophagic intervention [9, 10].

2. The molecular mechanism of autophagy

During macro-autophagy the formation of autophagosomes, representing double enveloped vesicles that enable the engulfment of targeted long-lived molecules and other cellular complexes from the remaining cytosol, are accomplished [11]. The following fusion with lysosomes containing proteolytic enzymes, i.e., the formation of autophagolysosomes, allows final degradation and reprocessing of their content [12]. The formation of the autophagosome is initiated by the phagopore assembly site (PAS) where autophagy-related (ATG) proteins are then recruited [13]. Particularly, the substantial work of the Nobel Prize laureate Ohsumi of ATG proteins in yeast has expedited our knowledge about the formation of the autophagosomes [14]. So far, 20 ATG proteins have been uncovered in mammalians that are activated during formation, enlargement, and closure of the autophagosome in a specific order. The process of autophagy has been categorized into several steps involving the ATG1/ULK kinase complex (initiation), the ATG12 conjugation system (nucleation), the ATG8/LC3 conjugation/deconjugation system (elongation), the phosphatidyl-inositol 3-kinase complex (maturation), and the ATG9/ATG9L1 cycling system (degradation). Either tumor suppressor proteins or oncogenes resulting in activation or suppression, respectively, have been determined to control the process of autophagy [15]. Consistently, key regulators that participate in the initial phase of autophagosome formation are the nutrient-sensing serine/threonine kinase mammalian target of rapamycin (mTOR), the unc-51 like autophagy activating kinases (ULK1/ULK2), the Beclin-1 (BECN1) lipid kinase complex, and the ubiquitin-like conjugation system (**Figure 1**) [16–19]. As an overall major player, the mTOR multiprotein complex (mTORC) functions, comparable to p53, as a sensor for multiple kinds of stress signals which are of genotoxic and oxidative nature, particularly represented by reactive oxygen species (ROS), and nutrient levels such as energy, amino acids, glucose, or growth factors [19, 20]. The integration of these signals by mTOR beside autophagy also serves for the regulation of various other cellular functions such as translation, cell cycle, microtubule organization, or lipid biogenesis [21]. The mTOR complex subsequently inhibits the ATG13-ULK-FIP200 complex, consisting of ATG13, ULK1 (ATG1), and the focal adhesion kinase interacting protein of 200 kD (FIP200), which is necessary to initiate phagopore formation [22–24]; frequently, nutrient starvation-induced autophagy involves the formation of this complex. Further reports however, also noticed mTOR-mediated downregulation of the p53 family member p73 entailing the transcriptional activation of ATG5, ATG7, and UVRAG genes [25, 26]. Together with the ATG13-ULK-FIP200 complex, mTOR binds to the haplo-insufficient tumor suppressor protein Beclin-1 (ATG6) that organizes the phagopore formation and subsequently elongation and maturation of the autophagosome in a concerted action with various interacting proteins [27, 28]. For this purpose, Beclin-1 forms the Vps34 core complex consisting of Vps15 and class III phosphatidylinositol 3-kinase (PIKC3) that enables the generation of phosphatidylinositol 3-phosphate (PI3P) [28, 29]. Due to death associated protein kinase (DAPK)-mediated phosphorylation, Beclin-1 is not only controlling

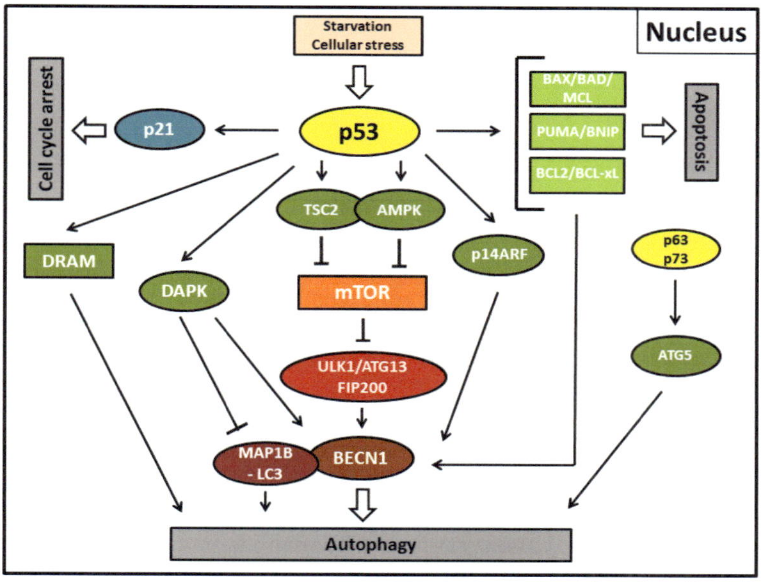

Figure 1.
Nuclear p53-mediated transcription-dependent autophagy, apoptosis and cell cycle arrest in response to stress conditions. By upregulation of tuberous sclerosis complex 2 (TSC2) or phosphatase and tensin homolog (PTEN; not shown), or AMP-activated protein kinase (AMPK) or its activators sestrins (not shown) p53 prevailingly attenuates mammalian target of rapamycin (mTOR) and the unc-51 like autophagy activating kinase 1 (ULK1) complex (consisting of autophagy-related gene 13 (ATG13) and the focal adhesion kinase interacting protein of 200 kD (FIP200)) as the autophagic canonical pathway. ULK-1 then interacts with Beclin-1 (BECN1) to initiate autophagosome formation. A shortcut for activation of autophagy involves damage-regulated autophagy modulator (DRAM), death associated protein kinase (DAPK), or autophagy-related gene 5 (ATG5) upregulation by the p53-family members, p63 and p73, or disruption of BCL2-family-or alternate reading frame protein product of the CDKN2A locus (p14ARF)-mediated release of BECN1 inhibition. In addition to autophagy, DRAM and p63/p73 are able to activate apoptosis. Arrowlines, upregulation or activation by indicated proteins; double arrow, major pathway activity. p53-mediated upregulation of the cyclin-dependent kinase inhibitor 1 (p21) enforces cell-cycle arrest. This figure is used under the terms and conditions of the creative commons attribution (CC BY) license (http://creativecommons.org/licenses/by/4.0/) derived from Mrakovcic and Fröhlich [57].

autophagy but found as a general regulator of lysosomes and endosome formation during membrane trafficking [30]. Further maturation of autophagosomes involves the interaction of the PI3P-binding proteins WIPI 1/2 with ATG12-ATG5-ATG16L and LC3-phosphatidylethanolamine (LC3-PE) complexes, both representing ubiquitin-like conjugation systems [4, 18, 31]. LC3 (microtubule-associated protein 1A/1B-light chain 3) and p62/Sequestosome-1 are two markers that are regularly employed for documenting autophagic flux as they are involved in the maturation of autophagosomes [32]. While LC3-I is processed to LC3-II, the scaffold protein p62 interacts with LC3 via its LC3-binding motif and seems to have a role in selectively guiding ubiquitinated proteins toward the autophagosome via its ubiquitin-binding domain [33]; thus, p62 levels decease during the induction of autophagy and have been found moreover to regulate protein deacetylation and is associated with tumorigenesis [34–36]. Autophagosome-lysosome fusion that requires the trans-membrane protein LAMP2 and small Rab GTPases, finally permits hydrolase and cathepsin-mediated processing of the autophagosome content [37, 38].

2.1 Positive regulation of p53-mediated autophagy

The tumor suppressor protein and transcription factor p53, which represents a “guardian” of the cell, has a fundamental role in the regulation of cell integrity and homeostasis and consequently in tumor defense. It coordinates cellular responses such as cell cycle arrest, apoptosis, senescence, metabolism, differentiation, angiogenesis, and even modulates autophagy. Among a multitude of other post-translational modifications, acetylation assists the master regulator to sense and integrate a variety of endogenous and exogenous cellular stress signals such as DNA damage, epigenetic alterations due to DNA methylation, genotoxicity, hypoxia, oxidative stress, or oncogene activation [39, 40]. In response, p53, as a central transcription factor translocates to the nucleus by detaching from the E3 ubiquitin ligase, mouse double minute 2 homolog (MDM2), and modulates the expression of multiple downstream target genes that regulate processes such as cell cycle progression and cell death [41, 42]. In appropriate conditions, p53 induces apoptosis by transactivating, i.e., transcriptional activation of pro-apoptotic genes or in the cytoplasm by direct interaction with anti-apoptotic proteins located in the mitochondrial membrane [43].

Several signaling pathways involving the transactivational activity of p53—in normal as well as cancer cells regulate autophagy in the classical canonical mTOR pathway as specified in the previous chapter (**Figure 1**) [44]. As pro-autophagic factors emanating from p53, these pathways involve on the one hand the tumor suppressor proteins tuberous sclerosis complex 2 (TSC2) and phosphatase and tensin homolog (PTEN), and on the other hand the nutrient energy sensor AMP-activated protein kinase (AMPK) or its activators sestrins 1 and 2 [45–47]. A further path that bypasses mTOR and can directly modulate p53 stress-activated signal transduction, is damage-regulated autophagy modulator (DRAM) that can activate the autophagic as well as apoptotic program [48]. As a protein located in the lysosome, it can intervene at different steps of autophagosome formation [49]. Furthermore, by either upregulating pro-apoptotic protein expression (BAX, BAD, BNIP3, or PUMA) or downregulating anti-apoptotic protein expression (BCL-2, BCL-xL and MCL-1) of the B-cell Lymphoma-2 (BCL-2) family, p53 can enforce dual activation of autophagy and apoptosis [50, 51]. In the inactivated state these proteins directly interact with the BH3 domain of BECLIN-1 and block the direct activation of BECLIN-1-dependent autophagy [52, 53]. Direct interaction of the nuclear full-length form of p53-modulated tumor suppressor protein p14ARF (an alternate reading frame protein of the CDKN2A locus) with the BCL-xL protein is a further similar mechanism promoting the induction of autophagy although the predominant role of p14ARF seems to stabilize p53 to protect the cell against hyperproliferative growth and associated activation of oncogenes [54, 55]. Additionally, p53-elicited upregulation of DAPK has been reported to result in autophagic activation either by DAPK-mediated phosphorylation of Beclin-1 that blocks its degradation by BCL-2/BCL-xL, or by impeding the anti-autophagic LC3-interacting MAP1B protein [30, 56].

2.2 Negative regulation of p53-mediated autophagy

Beyond the nuclear-based transactivating pro-autophagic effects mediated by p53, additional inhibitory anti-autophagic responses related to cytoplasm-localized p53 protein have been uncovered by Tasdemir et al. in the past 10 years (**Figure 2**) [58]. While the transactivation-dependent nuclear autophagic response of p53 is stimulated by stress induction, the cytoplasmic blockage of autophagic induction is a steady-state function that is present under physiological conditions and seems to engage direct protein interaction. This cytoplasm-mediated inhibition of autophagy was also characterized to activate the canonical p53-AMPK-mTOR signaling cascade. In contrast to transcription-dependent pathway, however, the positive autophagic regulator AMP-dependent kinase is inhibited by p53 which

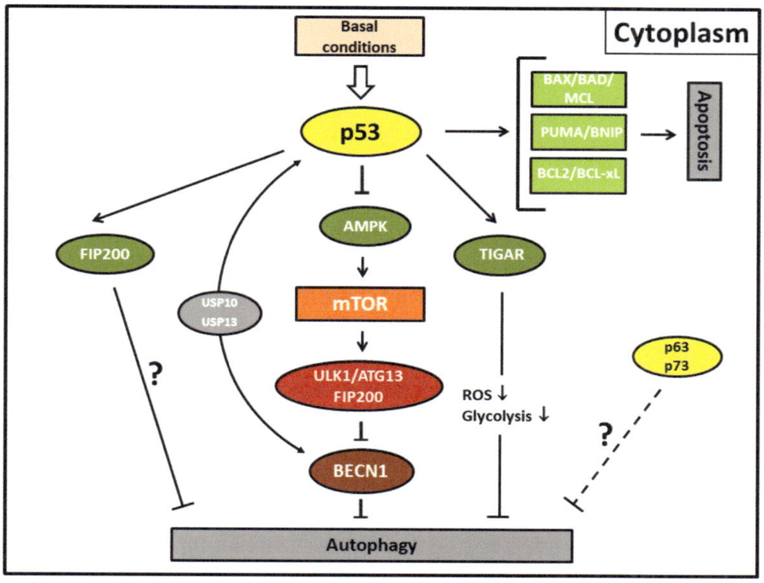

Figure 2.
Cytoplasmic p53-mediated transcription-independent autophagy (under physiological conditions) and apoptosis. By direct inhibition, wildtype p53-protein inactivates AMPK-mTOR-ULK1 transduced autophagy leading to BECN1 degradation. Similarly, BECN1 degradation can also be directly mediated by the ubiquitin-specific peptidases USP10 and USP13. Further inhibitory functions for autophagy can be mediated by TP53-induced glycolysis and apoptosis regulator (TIGAR) following the down-regulation of glycolysis and the suppression of reactive oxygen species (ROS) formation. Also, p63/p73 has been reported to presumably exert transcription-independent disruption of autophagy (dashed line); fork symbols, inhibition; arrowlines, activation by indicated proteins; downward arrow, downregulation. For abbreviations, see **Figure 1**. *This figure is used under the terms and conditions of the creative commons attribution (CC BY) license (http://creativecommons.org/licenses/by/4.0/) derived from Mrakovcic and Fröhlich [57].*

in turn activates mTOR [59]. Accordingly, either pharmacological interference, depletion of basal p53 levels, or p53 variants that possess a genetically modified nuclear export domain rendered cells more resistant toward metabolic stress through elevated autophagy. The underlying obscure mechanism that is found not only in mammalians but also in nematodes could involve direct binding of p53 to FIP200 (ATG17) as experimentally evidenced [60]. Negative regulation of autophagy by cytoplasmic p53 has been also linked to its target gene TIGAR (TP53-induced glycolysis and apoptosis regulator) that suppresses glycolysis and ROS generation when the cell is exerted to stress [61]. Nevertheless, although TIGAR mediates ROS-mediated induction of autophagy, it is not a likely candidate for the above described mechanism but rather represents an alternative path since it does not inhibit mTOR obviously. A similar but also unclear anti-autophagic mechanism could be verified in embryonal carcinoma cells, where p53-Beclin-1 interaction facilitated Beclin-1 ubiquitination and subsequent degradation, which could be de-activated by depletion of p53 [62]. Another report identified Beclin-1 as a regulator of de-ubiquitination of p53 which was mediated by USP10 and USP13 ubiquitin-specific peptidases [63]. This mechanism might therefore also relate to the previously mentioned Beclin-1-induced autophagy which enables bidirectional dual activation of apoptosis and autophagy [64].

2.3 Regulation of autophagy in p53-inactivated cells

p53 is one of the most frequently inactivated tumor suppressor genes in human tumors [65]. Particularly, single point mutations that provoke a loss of p53 function were documented that in several cases apply a dominant-negative effect to the remaining non-mutant allele thereby enhancing their oncogenic effect [41, 66, 67]. Often, such p53 variants result in increased genomic instability, attenuated chemotherapeutic success and a poor prognosis for patients [68]. One of the underlying reasons therefore could be that many tumor-derived p53 variants also inactivate cytoprotective or cytotoxic autophagy [69–71]. Nevertheless, although nucleus-based transcription-dependent autophagy might be shut down in these cases, cytoplasm-induced activation of the autophagic program might still be available, due to p53-deficiency or functional inactivation. Interestingly, the studies of Morselli et al. demonstrated that several tumor-derived mutants of p53 that reside in the cytoplasm are still able to block autophagic induction, presumably by direct protein interaction [70]. Such experiments underline the significance why it is meaningful to discriminate p53 mutant variants with regard to their potential effects. This finding also highlights the role of context-dependent autophagy during tumorigenesis as disabled autophagy by mutant p53 was found to prolong tumor cell survival while it inactivated its tumor suppressor function. Thus, increased proliferation of pancreas and breast cancer cells could be uncovered in a report that confirmed inhibition of autophagy by mutant gain-of-function p53 proteins. This counteractivity was evidenced by stimulation of AMPK-mTOR genes with concomitant downregulation of Beclin-1, DRAM, ATG12, and sestrin genes [72].

Various investigations found also a counter-acting surveillance mechanism between autophagy and since as mutant p53 blocks autophagic induction in one way but autophagy can stimulate the sequestering of mutant p53 in order to suppress tumorigenesis in the other way. Mechanistically, this mutual crosstalk is translated by the regulatory actions of the two suppressor genes Beclin-1 and p53 on autophagy as specified in the previous chapter [63]. While p53 exerts control on Beclin-1 via the canonical autophagic pathway, Beclin-1 also directly regulates p53 via controlling its deubiquitination activity which explains the mirrored effect on the phenotype of p53- and Beclin-1 ablated mice [73]. Additionally, with respect to Beclin-1 mediated autophagy, further reports documented the possibility of autophagic activation via the tumor suppressor protein p14ARF in p53-silenced or -inhibited cells [74]. Studies using doxorubicin-treated p53-wildtype or -deficient (p53−/−) mouse embryonic fibroblasts furthermore verified that the p53 family members p63 and p73 can substitute the loss of p53 (**Figure 2**) [75]; this mechanism involved nucleus translocation of p63/p73 and the increased expression of an extensive network of ATG proteins, such as ATG4a, ATG4c, ULK1, ULK2, UVRAG, and ATG5. This finding might explain resistance in doxorubicin-mediated chemotherapeutic treatment of cancer tissues.

3. Histone deacetylases and histone deacetylase inhibitors

Histone acetylation by the families of histone acetylases (HATs) histone deacetylases (HDACs) are crucial epigenetic elements in the regulation of gene transcription of histone as well as non-histone proteins. HATs catalyze acetylation to lysine residues of proteins, which stimulates a relaxed transcriptionally accessible chromatin configuration, while HDACs facilitate their removal associated with a closed transcriptionally inaccessible chromatin structure [76, 77]. Acetylation of histones and non-histones not only interferes with gene expression but crucially governs cell signaling and cellular processes such as proliferation, differentiation, and programmed cell death [78]. Identified non-histone substrates to date are tumor suppressor proteins (e.g., p53, RUNX3), signaling mediators (e.g., STAT3, β-catenin, Smad7), steroid receptors (e.g., androgen, estrogen, SHP), transcriptional factors, and co-regulators (e.g., c-Myc, HMG, YY1, EKLF, E2F1, GATA factors, HIF-1α, MyoD, NF-κB, and FoxB3), as well as structural (e.g., cell motility proteins), chaperone proteins, and nuclear import proteins (e.g., α-tubulin, importin-α, Ku70, HSP90) [79].

Depending on function or structure, four classes (class I–IV) have been allocated that comprise 18 members of the HDAC family [80]. The "classical HDACs" contain classes I and II and are functionally dependent on zinc as co-factor, while class III HDACs include the sirtuin proteins (Sirt1-7; homology to yeast Sir2) and require NAD+ [81]. Nevertheless, HDACs also differ in subcellular localization, and expression pattern [78]. While class I HDACs are expressed ubiquitously as they are located in the cell nucleus providing them with superior enzymatic activity, class II HDACs possess restricted tissue-specific expression pattern. Thus, they have been subdivided into class IIa HDACs (HDAC4, 5, 7 and 9) which shuttle between nucleus and cytoplasm as well as class IIb HDACs (HDAC 6 and 10) that are located mostly in the cytoplasm [82]. SIRTs exhibit specific subcellular presence in the nucleus (Sirt1, 6 and 7), in the cytoplasm (Sirt2), or in mitochondria (Sirt3, 4 and 5) which is not interchangeable. HDAC11, the single less-well explored member of class IV HDACs, has narrowed tissue expression [83].

HDAC inhibitors (HDACi) have been explored as a new category of anticancer drugs that reverses epigenetic changes established by the deregulated activities of HDACs in hematological as well as solid cancers [84]. HDACi treatment induces transcriptional de-repression of genes that are eminent regulators of tumor cell activities such as cell cycle arrest, differentiation, and programmed cell death and even the expression and stability of oncoproteins [85]. HDACi categories encompass hydroxamic acids (hydroxamates), cyclic tetrapeptides, benzamides, electrophilic ketones, and aliphatic acids that include natural but also synthetic derivatives that exhibit different structures [84]. Favored representatives of the hydroxamates are SAHA (suberoylanilide hydroxamic acid, vorinostat, and Zolinza) which is a preferred derivative of naturally occurring trichostatin A (TSA) as well as the CBHA (m-carboxycinnamic acid bishydroxamate)-derived tubacin, LAQ-824 (dacinostat), LBH-589 (panobinostat), or PXD-101 (belinostat) [86–89]. The class I-selective FK-228 (romidepsin, FR901228, istodax) belongs to the group of cyclic tetrapeptides [90]. MS-275 (entinostat) and MGCD0103 (mocetinostat) exhibiting enhanced HDAC class I selectivity are members of benzamide-based HDACi [91, 92]. The minor effective class I- and IIa-specific HDACi, VPA (valproic acid), PBA (phenylbutyrate), NaB (sodium butyrate), or AN-9 (pivaloyloxymethyl butyrate) belong to the category of aliphatic acids [93, 94]. This classification mainly depends on the chemical structure of their zinc-binding group but in addition HDACi can also be subdivided into zinc-dependent, pan- or broad-spectrum inhibitors that inhibit all class I, II and IV HDACs in contrast to primarily class I-specific HDACi [95]. Representatives of pan-inhibitors are TSA, SAHA, LBH589, and PXD-101 while valproic acid and butyrate inhibit exclusively class I HDACs. MS-275 and depsipeptide inhibits only a few members of class I HDACs, respectively. To date, the HDAC6-specific inhibitor tubacin is the only representative of an isoform-specific HDACi [86]. With the exception of nicotinamide, no clinical useful SIRT inhibitors have been uncovered yet [96].

Clinical trials of single or combined treatments of several HDACi with diverse results have been or are in the progress of being tested in hematological and solid cancers (www.clinicaltrials.gov) [97, 98]. Up to now, exclusively the evaluation of pan-inhibitors have succeeded in the admittance of four licensed HDACi, namely, SAHA, panobinostat (LBH589), belinostat (PXD-101), and romidepsin (FK228) for the treatment of cutaneous T cell lymphoma, multiple myeloma, or peripheral T cell lymphoma, respectively [99–103]. Although preclinical studies using single treatment regimen of many HDACi were encouraging, almost all entities of solid tumors (e.g., ovarian, breast, renal, prostate, and head and neck cancer) lacked positive effects in phase II clinical trials [104, 105]. In addition, patients suffered from trivial (e.g., dehydration, anorexia, diarrhea) to toxic (e.g., cardiotoxicity, thrombocytopenia myelosuppression) non-selective side effects [85, 94, 106]. The reasons for these drawbacks are presently non-elucidated and were assumed to be due to a combination of failing blood vessel supply, endogenous molecular heterogeneity owing to epigenetic modifications, and the development of treatment resistance. In response, selective HDAC-specific inhibitors are being developed, that target only one or two isozymes [107]. The design of novel or improved specific inhibitors will allow the full exploration of individual functions of distinct HDAC activity and may furthermore provide improved therapeutic efficacy together with less toxicity.

4. Mechanisms of histone deacetylase inhibitor-induced cell death

Owing to the various posttranslational histone and non-histone protein acetylation targets, HDACi exert a multitude of anti-tumor effects that concern interference with growth, differentiation, migration, senescence, and death [108]. Although there may be tumor cell-type and HDACi-specific effects which are unclear presently, common mechanisms are shaping for different HDACi [85, 108]. Induction of apoptosis is by far the prevailing avenue of HDACi triggered cell death in transformed cells which is prepared by re-induction of cell cycle arrest and induction cell differentiation, e.g., by the downregulation of positive cell growth regulators [109–112]. G1 or G2 phase induced cell cycle arrest in the G1 or G2 phase can occur in a p53-dependent or -independent manner by stimulating the upregulation of (p21waf-1/cip1) expression which is a cyclin-dependent kinase (CDKN) inhibitor of cyclins D1/D2 [113–115]. As an underlying mechanism it is assumed that the inability to exit the cell cycle from unfinished mitosis might sensitize the activation of apoptosis due to compiled DNA damage such as double-strand breaks [116, 117]. HDACi-stimulated activation of the intrinsic (mitochondrial) pathway of apoptosis involves either down-regulation of anti-apoptotic genes (e.g., BCL-2, BCL-XL, XIAP, MCL-1, and survivin) or overexpression of pro-apoptotic genes (e.g., BAX, BAK) belonging to the B-cell Lymphoma-2 (BCL-2) family [113, 114, 118, 119]. In the extrinsic (death-receptor) pathway, HDACi predominantly re-establish the expression of death receptors such as DR4 and DR5, or their corresponding ligands (e.g., TRAIL, FAS, FAS-L, and TNF-alpha) [120–122]. Furthermore, also the induction of reactive oxygen species (ROS) by HDACi is a second important anticancer-mechanism that is also responsible for cell death induction and associated with DNA damage; presumably, ROS is scavenged in normal, but not in malignant cells due to the compiled expression of thioredoxin (TXN) which represents an endogenous cellular antioxidant [123]. HDACs have moreover been detected to control histone deacetylation at damaged DNA sites undergoing repair that involves DNA damage-related response proteins [95, 124–132]. Thus, only in tumor cells upregulated expression of a marker for DNA double strand breaks, H2AX, was detected, when these were treated with SAHA [117]. In this context also the induction of autophagy as a means to maintain genomic was noticed, for instance, following MSH2-regulated DNA mismatch repair deregulation upon HDAC6 inhibition. Cell signaling pathways that were shut down in cancer cells can be furthermore re-established by immediately modifying acetylation of non-histone proteins such as transcription factors (e.g., NF-κB, p53, and STATs) [79]. As a prominent example, half-life and stability of p53 was influenced by MDM2 E3-ligase in HDACi-treated H1299 carcinoma cells [42]. In this way also chaperone protein function and the regulation of stress response pathways in the endoplasmic reticulum can be achieved, which affects the removal of misfolded proteins but also interference with stability and expression of oncoproteins [111, 133]. Additional mechanisms of HDACi-regulated lethality in tumor cells were evidenced in the interference with migration- and invasion capability due to re-established expression of metastasis-related genes and in the disruption of angiogenesis by altering pro- and anti-angiogenic gene expression [134–136]. In recent years, autophagy as a form of programmed cell death was added to the list of further determinants of HDACi-mediated effects that impedes cellular growth in a range of tumor cells [137–140].

5. Mechanisms of HDACi-induced autophagic cell death

An impressive diversity of mechanisms have been uncovered in cancer cells that promote HDACi-elicited autophagy which include mostly attenuation of mTOR signaling that can occur in combination combined with increased expression of LC3, Beclin-1, or ATG and can be provoked by endoplasmic reticulum stress (reviewed in [57] and **Table 1** [141]). mTOR is a well-known regulator of the canonical pathway of autophagy involving the regulation of the ULK1 complex and Beclin-1. The pivotal role of mTOR attenuated by SAHA-treatment which reestablishes ULK1 function could be initially verified by our own studies and those of Gammoh et al. using endometrial sarcoma cells, and were subsequently reiterated in many studies [71, 142]. It should be noticed that HDACi-induced autophagy is frequently accompanied by the additional induction of apoptosis.

Further predominant mechanisms of autophagic induction involve ROS accumulation, p21 upregulation, NF-κB hyperacetylation, and sirtuin-mediated acetylation of p53 [143–146]. In addition to mTOR downregulation, substantial intracellular ROS production interfering with mitochondrial function and energy metabolism has been demonstrated to facilitate SAHA-induced autophagy in tumor cells. ROS-induced autophagy can go along with additional increased expression of cathepsin D, a lysosomal protease, or decreased expression of TRX, representing its substrate and/or activation of the mitogen activated protein kinases ERK1/2 and JNK [143, 147]. Generally, enzymes related to energy metabolism, anti-oxidative stress and cellular redox control have been entangled by a proteomic study involving SAHA-administered Jurkat T-leukemia cells [147]. Cell cycle arrest, differentiation, and autophagy due to upregulated p21 expression were caused by treatment of PC-3 M and HL-60 cells with HDACi SAHA and H40 [148]. The same mechanism could be elicited by adding the novel HDACi, MRJF4, to prostate cancer cells autophagy [144]. As a further cause of SAHA/MS-275-induced autophagy in PC3 prostate cancer cells, re-activation of NF-κB associated target genes due to hyperacetylation of NF-κB RELA/p65, or downsizing of pERK/NF-κB signaling together with upregulated p21 expression, were described; however, the exact mechanism remains obscure [146].

Individual studies also noted nuclear translocation of the apoptosis inducing factor (AIF), apoptosome inactivation, FoxO1-stimulated expression, upregulation of DAPK or Nrf2, and p53-deficiency as regulatory mechanisms in HDACi-induced autophagy [71, 146, 149–153]. Thus, apoptosis, necrosis or autophagy were triggered in malignant rhabdoid tumor cells in response to FK228 (depsipeptide) treatment and upon silencing of the apoptosis inducing factor (AIF) that translocates into the nucleus for caspase-induced death, autophagy was suppressed as supported by transmission electron microscopy and LC3 measurements [149]. Following the blockage of the mitochondrial pathway of apoptosis by deleting caspase-9 or Apaf-1

Molecular mechanism	Additional mechanism	HDACi	Cell type	Ref.
mTOR inhibition	Increased p21 expression	SAHA	ESS-1	[156]
	Increase of LC3 expression; activation of ULK-1 complex	SAHA	MEFs, T98G glioblastoma	[142]
	Beclin-1 upregulation	SAHA, butyrate	HelaS3	[157]
	Induction of ER stress response	SAHA, OSU-HDAC42	HCC, Hep3B, HepG2	[158]
	ROS accumulation via Cat D, repression of TRX; BECN1 and ATG-7 upregulation.	SAHA	Jurkat T-leukemia	[147]
	BECN1 protein upregulation. and p62 downregulation	SAHA	Glioblastoma stem cells	[159]
	CASP and CPN-1 activation; reduced ATG expression*	MGCD0103	Primary CLL	[160]
	Increased ATG5 expression	Apicidin	Salivary MEC	[161]
ROS accumulation	CathD upregulation and TRX repression	SAHA	K562, LAMA 84 CMLL	[143]
	Activation of MAPK proteins: ERK1/2 and JNK; LC3 and ATG12 upregulation	FK228+ bortezomib	Gastric carcinoma (GC)	[162]
	p38 MAPK switch to apoptosis; ERK activation	M-275	HCT116	[163]
p21 $^{CIP/WAF1}$ upregulation	–	SAHA, H40	PC-3 M, HL-60	[148]
	Downregulation of pERK/ NF-κB signaling	MRJF4	PC3	[144]
NF-κB Hyper-acetylation	Induction of NF-κB target genes	SAHA, MS-275	PC3	[146]
AIF nucleus translocation	–	FK228	MRT	[149]
Apoptosome inactivation	Independent of p53; Deletion of Apaf-1/Casp-9	LAQ824, LBH589	Eμ-myc lymphomas	[152]
FoxO1 transcription	ATG expression; mTOR suppression via SESN3	SAHA, TSA	HepG2, HCT116	[150]
DAPK upregulation	–	LBH589	HCT116	[151]
Nrf2 upregulation	mTOR suppression via miR-129-3p	–	–	[153]
ATG7 acetylation*	Autophagy interactome acetylation; increased mitochondrial mass and ROS formation	SAHA, TSA, LBH589, JQ2	Megakaryoblastic leukemia	[154]
ATG gene upregulation*	Independent of p53 acetylation	Tenovin-6	CLL	[155]

Molecular mechanism	Additional mechanism	HDACi	Cell type	Ref.
p53 acetylation	Increased p53-dependent cell cycle arrest and apoptosis	Sirtinol	MCF-7	[145]
	p53 activation. by reducing MDM2 expression; cell cycle arrest and apodosis	MHY2256	MCF-7	[164]
p53-deficiency	mTOR inhibition	SAHA	ESS-1	[165]

*Leads to inhibition of autophagy; AVO (acidic vesicular organelles); (−), unknown or not determined. *

Table 1.
Mechanisms of HDACi-induced autophagic cell death.

or in Eμ-lymphomas the autophagic pathway was activated by the HDACi LAQ824 and LBH589 as evidenced morphologically and biochemically [152]. SAHA and TSA-induced autophagic cell survival via the transcription factor FoxO1 in HepG2 and HCT116 cells was furthermore mediated by sestrin 3 (SESN3)-induced mTOR inhibition and increased ATG protein expression [150]. Protein interaction or phosphorylation of the MAPK-interacting calcium- or calmodulin-regulated DAPK at serine 308 in HCT116 colon cancer cells, rather than its enzymatic function, moreover stimulated LBH589-induced autophagy [151]. Recently, even microRNA-mediated regulation of mTOR involving the transcription factor Nrf2 (nuclear factor erythroid 2 like-2) was implicated in HDACi-induced autophagy [153]. HDACi-induced Nrf2 mRNA and protein expression thereby promoted augmented transcription of miR-129-3p which facilitated mTOR attenuation. Nonetheless, even HDACi-mediated suppression of autophagy could be documented in two studies. Negative regulation of HDACi-mediated autophagy but upregulation of autophagic flux could be induced in myeloid-leukemic cells treated with valproic acid, SAHA, TSA, panobinostat, or JQ2 by acetylation and decreased expression of ATG7, a protein important for fusion of peroxisomal and vacuolar membranes [154]. Additionally, increased ATG expression following treatment with sirtuin inhibitor tenovin-6 provoked autophagic suppression in chronic lymphocytic leukemia (CLL) cells which was evident by upregulated genes of the autophagic-lysosomal pathway and LC3-II/p62 [154, 155].

6. HDACi-induced autophagy mediated by p53

p53 as the first described representative subjected non-histone protein acetylation can in response to stress positively as well as negatively regulate cell cycle arrest, senescence as well as apoptosis and autophagy [39, 40]. Acetylated residues attached by distinct HAT-mediated acetylation can be detected for p53 at distinct sites that could not only affect DNA binding and thereby its transactivational ability but also coactivator recruitment and/or its stability via proteasomal degradation [166–168]. For example, HDAC1-specific inhibition allows p53 to stay in an accessible state associated with transcriptional activity [169]. Furthermore, by mutating a combination of C-terminal sites that undergo acetylation p53-dependent transcription of p21 can be eliminated [170]. Nevertheless, the exact modalities of these mechanisms still need clarification. As previously specified, HDACi-mediated apoptosis that is commonly escorted by p21-mediated cell cycle arrest and ROS generation, has been documented as the most frequently encountered form of HDACi-triggered cell death [112, 119]. However, since transcription of pro-apoptotic genes, such as Bax, Noxa, and Puma, by p53 may be limited by posttranslational acetylation, the role of p53 in this relation is discussed. These assumptions are supported for example by the finding that p53-independent p21 induction and apoptosis upon HDACi administration and the anticancer effect of HDACi is not influenced by the mutational status of p53 in the tumor [109, 113]. Other reports in contrast verified p53 acetylation and stabilization in several tumor models in response to HDACi administration that presented cell cycle arrest and apoptosis [111, 171]. Conclusively, p53-dependent but also -independent signaling pathways may add to HDACi-mediated apoptotic processes and HDACi may induce p53, but do not unconditionally require p53 for providing anticancer effects. In recent time, the range of HDACi-exerted mechanisms resulting in cellular demise of cancer cells have been expanded by the induction of autophagic cell death which can alternatively or additionally to apoptosis activate autophagy (reviewed in [57, 141, 172] and **Table 1**). Also, involvement of posttranslational modification of the non-histone p53 has been linked to the control of HDACi-stimulated autophagy as evident from its key regulatory role in normal cells. This might of crucial advantage if tumor cells have developed resistance toward apoptotic cell death induction. Thus, experimental evidence from our studies of endometrial sarcoma (ESS) cells support a major regulatory function for p53 in directing cell death either toward HDACi-elicited apoptosis or autophagy [165].

In our model, the detection of HDAC2 overexpression in malignant endometrial stroma sarcoma cell lines led to the establishment of therapeutic SAHA treatment and the evaluation of its mechanism of action [173]. Significantly advanced cell death in MES-SA and ESS-1 cells was accompanied by previous p21-induced cell cycle arrest at the G1/S transition and reduced expression of HDAC2 and 7 [156, 173]. Either predominant caspase-dependent apoptotic (48%) or caspase-independent autophagic cell death (80%) was attested in SAHA-treated MES-SA and ESS cells after 24 h, respectively [156]. In line with the induction of the canonical pathway of autophagy, attenuated mTOR protein expression could be evidenced in ESS-1 cells in contrast to MES-SA cells [165]. Further screening of key regulatory molecules for apoptosis and for autophagy, upstream of mTOR, were performed to explain the differences in the modes of SAHA-induced cell death. This search uncovered entire absence of detectable p53 protein and lowered levels of PUMA protein in ESS-1 cells. Investigation of p53 gene and mRNA led to the detection of a novel nonsense mutation ($p53^{R213X}$) in the transactivating domain of p53 of ESS-1 cells that obviously provoked a degradation of the entire p53 transcript and could not be documented in MES-SA cells. Consistent with this finding, restoration of ESS-1 cells with a wild-type p53 variant restored induction of caspase-dependent apoptosis as supported by PUMA and caspase-9 upregulation as well as activation of the effector caspases-3 and -7 and final PARP-1 cleavage. Increased mTOR levels demonstrated the re-induction of basal autophagic flux in addition to apoptosis induction as verified by LC3 staining. Generalization of this finding could be obtained by several other p53-deficient tumor cell lines (such as PANC-1, Jurkat, HL-60, and U937) that are known to induce autophagy in response to SAHA and were supplied with wild-type p53.

We concluded that the molecular switch between SAHA-induced apoptosis and autophagy was thus mediated by the occurrence of functional p53 protein. Our experimental evidence thus underlines an overall major regulatory role for p53 not only in HDACi-mediated apoptosis but also in HDACi-stimulated autophagy (**Figure 3**) (reviewed in [57, 141]). As a consequence, p53-deficiency

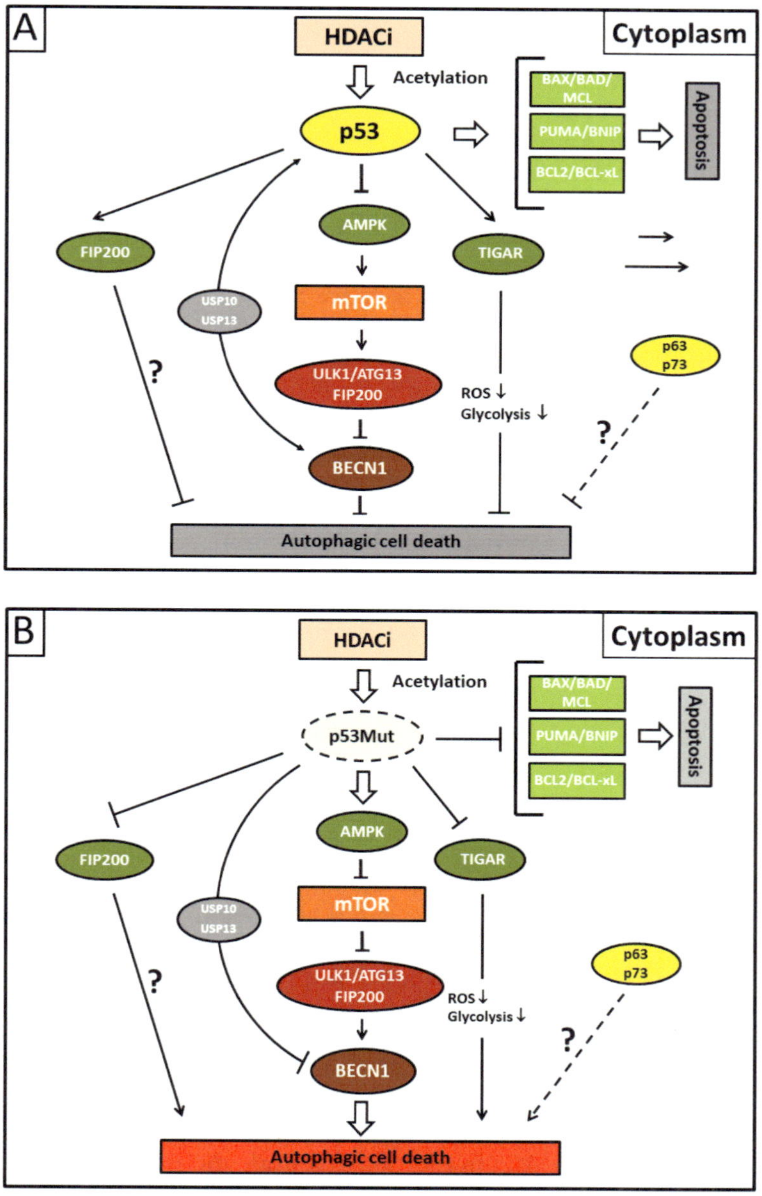

Figure 3.

Illustration depicting presumed mechanisms mediating SAHA-induced autophagy reflecting autophagic regulation by cytoplasmic mutant and wild-type p53. (A) Acetylated cytoplasmic p53 protein predominantly activates apoptotic cell death by direct binding to the BCL-2 family of pro-apoptotic proteins. Concomitantly, cytoplasmic p53 protein inhibits autophagic cell death by inducing Beclin-1 degradation via USP10/USP13 and/or inhibiting the AMPK-mTOR-ULK1 signaling pathway. It is unclear whether the canonical pathway is mediated by direct p53-FIP200 interaction or whether this represents an extra pathway. TIGAR inhibits autophagy by down-regulation of glycolysis and a suppression of ROS formation. The members of the p53 family, p63/p73, are also potential inhibitors of autophagy (dashed line). (B) Mutant p53 protein variants lose the ability of autophagic inhibition and apoptosis stimulation and activate autophagy. Fork symbols, inhibition; arrowlines, activation or interaction; double arrow, major pathway activity. This figure is used under the terms and conditions of the creative commons attribution (CC BY) license (http://creativecommons.org/licenses/by/4.0/) derived from Mrakovcic and Fröhlich [57].

could moreover explain apoptosis resistance as well predominant induction of HDACi-provoked autophagy in cancer cells. The presumptive negative regulation of autophagy by functional cytoplasmic p53 protein in SAHA-treated ESS-1 cells is moreover very consistent with the above discussed role of p53 as a dual regulator of autophagy by Tasdemir et al. [59]. Their findings convincingly describe nuclear p53 protein as an activator of transcription-dependent autophagy, in contrast to the inhibitory autophagic control by cytoplasmic p53 protein. In addition, by our report we link SAHA-induced acetylation of p53 to the mTOR signaling pathway which has been less evaluated to date, nonetheless, future experiments are needed to directly address this question.

In line with our experiments, the class III Sirt1 and 2-specific HDACi sirtinol, that affects acetylation of p53, has also been documented to determine HDACi-induced cell fate in several reports. For instance, p53 was entangled in balancing sirtinol-mediated apoptosis and autophagy in MCF-7 breast cancer cells [145]. Sirtinol treatment on the one hand preferentially induced predominant autophagy as shown by LC3-II upregulation, while addition of the autophagic inhibitor 3-methyladenine augmented cell cycle arrest and cytochrome C-triggered apoptotic cell death caused by increased BAX and diminished BCL-2 protein expression. In a similar experiment, inhibition by sirtinol and the novel SIRT1, -2, and -3 protein inhibitor, MHY2256, a similar phenotype that included cell cycle arrest and both types of programmed cell death could be provoked [164]. As a mechanistic explanation, SIRT1 and 2-induced acetylation of p53 at lysine 382 were found to inhibit ubiquitination of p53 via MDM2 which stabilized and increased its functional activity. MDM2-mediated degradation of p53 was also documented in MHY2256-treated Ishikawa cells that are derived from endometrial cancer which elicited activation of apoptosis together with autophagy as supported by elevated levels of p21, BAX and BCL-2, cytochrome C release, and cleaved PARP-1 [174].

7. Conclusions and perspectives

In recent times, epigenetic studies gained increasing significance in reports investigating the development of cancer. For this purpose, aberrant epigenetic patterns such as DNA methylation including the misguided expression of HDACs activity has been defined to some extent in many tumors which explains their selection as targets for anticancer therapy. Posttranslational modifications of histones and non-histones in the form of acetylation and deacetylation particularly enable pharmacological interference by different kind of inhibitors such as HDACi. The ability to sensitize apoptosis-resistant tumor cells by the disruption of autophagy was considered a promising route for cancer therapy as this process heightens the pro-apoptotic effects of HDACi. In addition to restrain the extents of tumor necrosis and inflammation however, autophagy might be required for the cancer cell to deal with metabolic stress and cytotoxicity during chemotherapy. Furthermore, by expediting the autophagic pathway in advanced stages of the cancer cell, autophagy may promote cell death by mostly non-elucidated mechanisms. Consistently, it is of pivotal importance to define the factors and mechanisms that influence the balance between HDACi-elicited apoptosis, autophagy or even necrosis in the cancer cell. In this regard, considerable research efforts are in progress to investigate the molecular pathways regulating HDACi-mediated cell death in tumor cells. The expansion of the knowledge about p53 as a mediator of apoptotic and autophagic cell death may as thus help to achieve progress not only in unraveling pathogenetic insights but also in the development of novel therapeutic strategies of such disease conditions as cancer.

Author details

Maria Mrakovcic[1,2] and Leopold F. Fröhlich[1*]

1 Department of Cranio-Maxillofacial Surgery, University of Münster, Germany

2 Department of Medical Microbiology, University of Münster, Germany

*Address all correspondence to: leopold.froehlich@ukmuenster.de

References

[1] Hanahan D, Weinberg RA. The hallmarks of cancer. Cell. 2000;**100**: 57-50

[2] Hanahan D, Weinberg RA. Hallmarks of cancer: The next generation. Cell. 2011;**144**:646-674

[3] Mariño G, Niso-Santano M, Baehrecke EH, Kroemer G. Self consumption: The interplay between autophagy and apoptosis. Nature Reviews. Molecular Cell Biology. 2014;**15**:81-94

[4] Mizushima N, Noda T, Yoshimori T, Tanaka Y, Ishii T, George MD, et al. A protein conjugation system essential for autophagy. Nature. 1998;**39**:395-398

[5] Yang Z, Klionsky DJ. Mammalian autophagy: Core molecular machinery and signaling regulation. Current Opinion in Cell Biology. 2010;**22**:124-131

[6] Choi AM, Ryter SW, Levine B. Autophagy in human health and disease. The New England Journal of Medicine. 2013;**368**:651-662

[7] Mathew R, Karantza-Wadsworth V, White E. Role of autophagy in cancer. Nature Reviews. Cancer. 2007;**7**:961-967

[8] He C, Klionsky DJ. Regulation mechanisms and signaling pathways of autophagy. Annual Review of Genetics. 2009;**43**:67-93

[9] Lopez G, Torres K, Liu J, Hernandez B, Young E, Belousov R, et al. Autophagic survival in resistance to histone deacetylase inhibitors: Novel strategies to treat malignant peripheral nerve sheath tumors. Cancer Research. 2011;**71**:185-196

[10] Rosenfeldt MT, Ryan KM. The role of autophagy in tumour development and cancer therapy. Expert Reviews in Molecular Medicine. 2009;**11**:e36

[11] Bento CF, Renna M, Ghislat G, Puri C, Ashkenazi A, Vicinanza M, et al. Mammalian autophagy: How does it work? Annual Review of Biochemistry. 2016;**85**:685-713

[12] Reggiori F, Ungermann C. Autophagosome maturation and fusion. Journal of Molecular Biology. 2017;**429**:486-496

[13] Rubinsztein DC, Shpilka T, Elazar Z. Mechanisms of autophagosome biogenesis. Current Biology. 2012;**22**:R29-R34

[14] Mizushima N, Yoshimori T, Ohsumi Y. The role of Atg proteins in autophagosome formation. Annual Review of Cell and Developmental Biology. 2011;**27**:107-132

[15] Maiuri MC, Tasdemir E, Criollo A, Morselli E, Vicencio JM, Carnuccio R, et al. Control of autophagy by oncogenes and tumor suppressor genes. Cell Death and Differentiation. 2009;**16**:87-93

[16] Jung CH, Ro SH, Cao J, Otto NM, Kim DH. mTOR regulation of autophagy. FEBS Letters. 2010;**584**:1287-1295

[17] Liang XH, Jackson S, Seaman M, Brown K, Kempkes B, Hibshoosh H, et al. Induction of autophagy and inhibition of tumorigenesis by Beclin 1. Nature. 1999;**402**:672-676

[18] Mizushima N, Sugita H, Yoshimori T, Ohsumi Y. A new protein conjugation system in human. The counterpart of the yeast Apg12p conjugation system essential for autophagy. The Journal of Biological Chemistry. 1998;**273**:33889-33892

[19] Noda T. Regulation of autophagy through TORC1 and mTORC1. Biomolecules. 2017;7:52

[20] Kim D, Sarbassov D, Ali S, King J, Latek R, Erdjument-Bromage H, et al. mTOR interacts with raptor to form a nutrient-sensitive complex that signals to the cell growth machinery. Cell. 2002;**110**:163-175

[21] Laplante M, Sabatini D. mTOR signaling. Cold Spring Harbor Perspectives in Biology. 2012;**4**:a011593

[22] Jung CH, Jun CB, Ro S, Kim Y, Otto NM, Cao J, et al. ULK-Atg13-FIP200 complexes mediate mTOR signaling to the autophagy machinery. Molecular Biology of the Cell. 2009;**20**:1992-2003

[23] Ganley IG, Lam DH, Wang J, Ding X, Chen S, Jiang X. ULK1.ATG13. FIP200 complex mediates mTOR signaling and is essential for autophagy. Journal of Biological Chemistry. 2009;**284**:12297-12305

[24] Kim J, Kundu M, Viollet B, Kun-Liang G. AMPK and mTOR regulate autophagy through direct phosphorylation of Ulk1. Nature Cell Biology. 2011;**13**:132-141

[25] Rosenbluth JM, Mays DJ, Pino MF, Tang LJ, Pietenpol JA. A gene signature-based approach identifies mTOR as a regulator of p73. Molecular and Cellular Biology. 2008;**28**:5951-5964

[26] Rosenbluth JM, Pietenpol JA. mTOR regulates autophagy-associated genes downstream of p73. Autophagy. 2009;**2**:1-7

[27] Maiuri M, Criollo A, Kroemer G. Crosstalk between apoptosis and autophagy within the Beclin 1 interactome. The EMBO Journal. 2010;**29**:515-516

[28] Liang XH, Jackson S, Seaman M, Brown K, Kempkes B, Hibshoosh H, et al. Induction of autophagy and inhibition of tumorigenesis by Beclin 1. Nature. 1999;**402**:1-5

[29] He C, Levine B. The Beclin 1 interactome. Current Opinion in Cell Biology. 2010;**22**:140-149

[30] Zalckvar E, Berissi H, Eisenstein MAK. Phosphorylation of Beclin 1 by DAP-kinase promotes autophagy by weakening its interactions with Bcl-2 and Bcl-XL. Autophagy. 2009;**5**:720-722

[31] Polson HE, de Lartigue J, Ridgen DJ, Reedijk M, Urbe S, Clague MJ, et al. Mammalian Atg18 (WIPI2) localizes to omegasome-anchored phagophores and positively regulates LC3 lipidation. Autophagy. 2010;**6**:506-522

[32] Bjørkøy G, Lamark T, Pankiv S, Øvervatn A, Brech ATJ. Monitoring autophagic degradation of p62/SQSTM1. Methods in Enzymology. 2009;**452**:181-197

[33] Seibenhener ML, Geetha T, Wooten MW. Sequestosome 1/p62—More than just a scaffold. FEBS Letters. 2007;**581**:175-179

[34] Mathew R, Karp CM, Beaudoin B, Vuong N, Chen G, Chen HY, et al. Autophagy suppresses tumorigenesis through elimination of p62. Cell. 2009;**137**:1062-1075

[35] Lahiri P, Schmidt V, Smole C, Kufferath I, Denk H, Strnad P, et al. P62/sequestosome-1 is indispensable for maturation and stabilization of Mallory-Denk bodies. PLoS One. 2016;**11**:e0161083

[36] Yang H, Ni HM, Guo F, Ding Y, Shi YH, Lahiri P, et al. Sequestosome 1/p62 protein is associated with autophagic removal of excess hepatic endoplasmic reticulum in mice. The Journal of Biological Chemistry. 2016;**29**:M116.739821

[37] Xie Z, Klionsky DJ. Autophagosome formation: Core machinery and adaptations. Nature Cell Biology. 2007;**9**:1102-1109

[38] Simonsen A, Tooze S. Coordination of membrane events during autophagy by multiple class III PI3-kinase complexes. The Journal of Cell Biology. 2009;**186**:773-782

[39] Vousden KH, Lane DP. p53 in health and disease. Nature Reviews. Molecular Cell Biology. 2007;**8**:275-283

[40] Gu W, Roeder RG. Activation of p53 sequence-specific DNA binding by acetylation of the p53 C-terminal domain. Cell. 1997;**90**:595-606

[41] Vousden KH, Lu X. Live or let die: The cell's response to p53. Nature Reviews. Cancer. 2002;**2**:594-604

[42] Tang Y, Zhao W, Chen Y, Zhao Y, Gu W. Acetylation is indispensable for p53 activation. Cell. 2008;**133**:612-626

[43] Chipuk JE, Green DR. Dissecting p53-dependent apoptosis. Cell Death and Differentiation. 2006;**13**:994-1002

[44] Galluzzi L, Morselli E, Kepp O, Maiuri MC, Kroemer G. Defective autophagy control by the p53 rheostat in cancer. Cell Cycle. 2010;**9**:250-255

[45] Arico S, Petiot A, Bauvy C, Dubbelhuis PF, Meijer AJ, Codogno P, et al. The tumor suppressor PTEN positively regulates macroautophagy by inhibiting the phosphatidylinositol 3-kinase/ protein kinase B pathway. The Journal of Biological Chemistry. 2001;**276**:35243-35246

[46] Feng Z. p53 regulation of the IGF-1/AKT/mTOR pathways and the endosomal compartment. Cold Spring Harbor Perspectives in Biology. 2010;**2**:a001057

[47] Budanov AV, Karin M. p53 target genes sestrin1 and sestrin2 connect genotoxic stress and mTOR signaling. Cell. 2008;**134**:451-460

[48] Crighton D, Wilkinson S, O'Prey J, Syed N, Smith P, Harrison PR, et al. DRAM, a p53-induced modulator of autophagy, is critical for apoptosis. Cell. 2006;**126**:121-134

[49] Crighton D, Wilkinson S, Ryan K. DRAM links autophagy to p53 and programmed cell death. Autophagy. 2007;**3**:72-74

[50] Maiuri M, Le Toumelin G, Criollo A, Rain J, Gautier F, Juin P, et al. Functional and physical interaction between Bcl-X(L) and a BH3-like domain in Beclin-1. The EMBO Journal. 2007;**26**:2527-2539

[51] Zalckvar E, Berissi H, Mizrachy L, Idelchuk Y, Koren I, Eisenstein M, et al. DAP-kinase mediated phosphorylation on the BH3 domain of beclin 1 promotes dissociation of beclin 1 from Bcl-XL and induction of autophagy. EMBO Reports. 2009;**10**:285-292

[52] Wang EY, Gang H, Aviv Y, Dhingra R, Margulets V, Kirshenbaum LA. p53 mediates autophagy and cell death by a mechanism contingent on Bnip3. Hypertension. 2013;**62**:70-77

[53] Pattingre S, Tassa A, Qu X, Garuti R, Liang X, Mizushima N, et al. Bcl-2 antiapoptotic proteins inhibit Beclin 1-dependent autophagy. Cell. 2005;**122**:927-939

[54] Pimkina J, Humbey O, Zilfou J, Jarnik M, Murphy M. ARF induces autophagy by virtue of interaction with Bcl-xl. The Journal of Biological Chemistry. 2009;**284**:2803-2810

[55] Budina-Kolomets A, Hontz RD, Pimkina J, Murphy ME. A conserved domain in exon 2 coding for the human and murine ARF tumor suppressor protein is required for autophagy induction. Autophagy. 2013;**9**:1553-1565

[56] Harrison B, Kraus M, Burch L, Stevens C, Craig A, Gordon-Weeks

P, et al. DAPK-1 binding to a linear peptide motif in MAP1B stimulates autophagy and membrane blebbing. The Journal of Biological Chemistry. 2008;**283**:9999-10014

[57] Mrakovcic M, Fröhlich LF. p53-mediated molecular control of autophagy in tumor cells. Biomolecules. 2018;**8**:E14

[58] Tasdemir E, Chiara Maiuri M, Morselli E, Criollo A, D'Amelio M, Djavaheri-Mergny M, et al. A dual role of p53 in the control of autophagy. Autophagy. 2008;**4**:810-814

[59] Tasdemir E, Maiuri MC, Galluzzi L, Vitale I, Djavaheri-Mergny M, D'Amelio M, et al. Regulation of autophagy by cytoplasmic p53. Nature Cell Biology. 2008;**10**:676-687

[60] Morselli E, Shen S, Ruckenstuhl C, Bauer M, Mariño G, Galluzzi L, et al. p53 inhibits autophagy by interacting with the human ortholog of yeast Atg17, RB1CC1/FIP200. Cell Cycle. 2011;**10**:2763-2769

[61] Bensaad K, Cheung EC, Vousden KH. Modulation of intracellular ROS levels by TIGAR controls autophagy. The EMBO Journal. 2009;**28**:3015-3026

[62] Tripathi R, Ash D, Shaha C. Beclin-1—p53 interaction is crucial for cell fate determination in embryonal carcinoma cells. Journal of Cellular and Molecular Medicine. 2014;**18**:2275-2286

[63] Liu J, Xia H, Kim M, Xu L, Li Y, Zhang L, et al. Beclin1 controls the levels of p53 by regulating the deubiquitination activity of USP10 and USP13. Cell. 2011;**147**:223-234

[64] Yousefi S, Perozzo R, Schmid I, Ziemiecki A, Schaffner T, Scapozza L, et al. Calpain-mediated cleavage of Atg5 switches autophagy to apoptosis. Nature Cell Biology. 2006;**8**:1124-1132

[65] Muller PAJ, Vousden KH. P53 mutations in cancer. Nature Cell Biology. 2013;**15**:2-8

[66] Dittmer D, Pati S, Zambetti G, Chu S, Teresky AK, Moore M, et al. Gain of function mutations in p53. Nature Genetics. 1993;**4**:42-46

[67] Santoro R, Strano S, Blandino G. Transcriptional regulation by mutant p53 and oncogenesis. Sub-Cellular Biochemistry. 2014;**85**:91-103

[68] Liu J, Ma Q, Zhang M, Wang X, Zhang D, Li W, et al. Alterations of TP53 are associated with a poor outcome for patients with hepatocellular carcinoma: Evidence from a systematic review and metaanalysis. European Journal of Cancer. 2012;**48**:2328-2338

[69] Cordani M, Butera G, Pacchiana R, Donadelli M. Molecular interplay between mutant p53 proteins and autophagy in cancer cells. Biochimica et Biophysica Acta, Reviews on Cancer. 2017;**1867**:19-28

[70] Morselli E, Tasdemir E, Maiuri MC, Galluzzi L, Kepp O, Criollo A, et al. Mutant p53 protein localized in the cytoplasm inhibits autophagy. Cell Cycle. 2008;**7**:3056-3061

[71] Fröhlich LF, Mrakovcic M, Smole C, Zatloukal K. Molecular mechanism leading to SAHA-induced autophagy in tumor cells: Evidence for a p53-dependent pathway. Cancer Cell International. 2016;**16**:68

[72] Cordani M, Oppici E, Dando I, Butturini E, Dalla Pozza E, Nadal-Serrano M, et al. Mutant p53 proteins counteract autophagic mechanism sensitizing cancer cells to mTOR inhibition. Molecular Oncology. 2016;**10**:1008-1029

[73] Qu X, Yu J, Bhagat G, Furuya N, Hibshoosh H, Troxel A, et al. Promotion of tumorigenesis by

heterozygous disruption of the beclin 1 autophagy gene. The Journal of Clinical Investigation. 2003;**112**:1809-1820

[74] Abida WM, Gu W. p53-dependent and p53-independent activation of autophagy by ARF. Cancer Research. 2008;**68**:352-357

[75] Kenzelmann Broz D, Mello SS, Bieging KT, Jiang D, Dusek RL, Brady CA, et al. Global genomic profiling reveals an extensive p53-regulated autophagy program contributing to key p53 responses. Genes and Development. 2013;**27**:1016-1031

[76] Marmorstein R, Roth SY. Histone acetyltransferases: Function, structure, and catalysis. Current Opinion in Genetics and Development. 2001;**11**:155-161

[77] Gray SG, Ekstro TJ. The human histone deacetylase family. Experimental Cell Research. 2001;**262**:75-83

[78] de Ruijter AJ, van Gennip AH, Caron HN, Kemp S, van Kuilenburg AB. Histone deacetylases (HDACs): Characterization of the classical HDAC family. The Biochemical Journal. 2003;**370**:737-749

[79] Spange S, Wagner T, Heinzel T, Krämer OH. Acetylation of non-histone proteins modulates cellular signalling at multiple levels. The International Journal of Biochemistry and Cell Biology. 2009;**41**:185-198

[80] Yang XJ, Edward S. The Rpd3/Hda1 family of lysine deacetylases: From bacteria and yeast to mice and men. Nature Reviews. Molecular Cell Biology. 2009;**9**:206-218

[81] Haigis MC, Guarente LP. Mammalian sirtuins—Emerging roles in physiology, aging, and calorie restriction. Genes and Development. 2006;**20**:2913-2921

[82] Yang X, Gregoire S. Class II histone deacetylases: From sequence to function, regulation, and clinical implication. Molecular and Cellular Biology. 2005;**25**:2873-2884

[83] Gao L, Cueto MA, Asselbergs F, Atadja P. Cloning and functional characterization of HDAC11, a novel member of the human histone deacetylase family. The Journal of Biological Chemistry. 2002;**277**:25748-25755

[84] Dokmanovic M, Clarke C, Marks PA. Histone deacetylase inhibitors: Overview and perspectives. Molecular Cancer Research. 2007;**5**:981-989

[85] Eckschlager T, Plch J, Stiborova M, Hrabeta J. Histone deacetylase inhibitors as anticancer drugs. International Journal of Molecular Sciences. 2017;**18**:1414

[86] Haggarty SJ, Koeller KM, Wong JC, Grozinger CM, Schreiber SL. Domain-selective small-molecule inhibitor of histone deacetylase 6 (HDAC6)-mediated tubulin deacetylation. Proceedings of the National Academy of Sciences of the United States of America. 2003;**100**:4389-4394

[87] Richon V, Emiliani S, Verdin E, Webb Y, Breslow R, Rifkind RA, et al. A class of hybrid polar inducers of transformed cell differentiation inhibits histone deacetylases. Proceedings of the National Academy of Sciences of the United States of America. 1998;**95**:3003-3007

[88] Coffey DC, Kutko MC, Glick RD, Butler LM, Heller G, Rifkind RA, et al. The Histone deacetylase inhibitor, CBHA, inhibits growth of human neuroblastoma xenografts in vivo, alone and synergistically with all-trans retinoic acid. Cancer Research. 2001;**61**:3591-3594

[89] Plumb JA, Finn PW, Williams RJ, Bandara MJ, Romero MR, Watkins CJ, et al. Pharmacodynamic response

and inhibition of growth of human tumor xenografts by the novel histone deacetylase inhibitor PXD101. Molecular Cancer Therapeutics. 2003;**2**:721-728

[90] Furumai R, Matsuyama A, Kobashi N, Lee K, Nishiyama M, Nakajima H, et al. FK228 (depsipeptide) as a natural prodrug that inhibits class I histone deacetylases. Cancer Research. 2002;**62**:4916-4921

[91] Maggio SC, Rosato RR, Kramer LB, Dai Y, Rahmani M, Paik DS, et al. The histone deacetylase inhibitor MS-275 interacts synergistically with fludarabine to induce apoptosis in human leukemia cells. Cancer Research. 2004;**64**:2590-2600

[92] Boumber Y, Younes A, Garcia-Manero G. Mocetinostat (MGCD0103): A review of an isotype-specific histone deacetylase inhibitor. Expert Opinion on Investigational Drugs. 2011;**20**:823-829

[93] Minucci S, Zhu P, Kramer O, Schimpf A, Giavara S, Sleeman JP, et al. Valproic acid defines a novel class of HDAC inhibitors inducing differentiation of transformed cells. The EMBO Journal. 2001;**20**:6969-6978

[94] Rasheed WK, Johnstone RW, Prince HM. Histone deacetylase inhibitors in cancer therapy. Expert Opinion on Investigational Drugs. 2017;**16**:659-678

[95] Li Y, Seto E. HDACs and HDAC inhibitors in cancer development and therapy. Cold Spring Harbor Perspectives in Medicine. 2016;**6**:a026831

[96] Avalos JL, Bever KM, Wolberger C. Mechanism of sirtuin inhibition by nicotinamide : Altering the NAD+ cosubstrate specificity of a Sir2 enzyme. Molecular Cell. 2005;**17**:855-868

[97] Wagner JM, Hackanson B, Lübbert M, Jung M. Histone deacetylase (HDAC) inhibitors in recent clinical trials for cancer therapy. Clinical Epigenetics. 2010;**1**:117-136

[98] Tan J, Cang S, Ma Y, Petrillo RL, Liu D. Novel histone deacetylase inhibitors in clinical trials as anti-cancer agents. Journal of Hematology and Oncology. 2010;**3**:1-13

[99] Duvic M, Vu J. Update on the treatment of cutaneous T-cell lymphoma (CTCL): Focus on vorinostat. Biologics. 2007;**1**:377

[100] Duvic M, Talpur R, Ni X, Zhang C, Hazarika P, Kelly C, et al. Phase 2 trial of oral vorinostat (suberoylanilide hydroxamic acid, SAHA) for refractory cutaneous T-cell lymphoma (CTCL). Blood. 2007;**109**:31-39

[101] Bertino EM, Otterson GA. Romidepsin: A novel histone deacetylase inhibitor for cancer. Expert Opinion on Investigational Drugs. 2011;**20**:1151-1158

[102] Rashidi A, Cashen AF. Belinostat for the treatment of relapsed or refractory peripheral T-cell lymphoma. Future Oncology. 2015;**11**:1659-1664

[103] Greig SL. Panobinostat: A review in relapsed or refractory multiple myeloma. Targeted Oncology. 2016;**11**:107-114

[104] Slingerland M, Guchelaar HJ, Gelderblom H. Histone deacetylase inhibitors: An overview of the clinical studies in solid tumors. Anti-Cancer Drugs. 2014;**25**:140-149

[105] Rasheed W, Bishton M, Johnstone RW, Prince HM. Histone deacetylase inhibitors in lymphoma and solid malignancies. Expert Review of Anticancer Therapy. 2008;**8**:413-432

[106] O'Connor OA, Heaney ML, Schwartz L, Richardson S, Willim R, MacGregor-Cortelli B, et al. Clinical

experience with intravenous and oral formulations of the novel histone deacetylase inhibitor suberoylanilide hydroxamic acid in patients with advanced hematologic malignancies. Journal of Clinical Oncology. 2017;**24**:166-173

[107] Balasubramanian S, Verner E, Buggy JJ. Isoform-specific histone deacetylase inhibitors: The next step ? Cancer Letters. 2009;**280**:211-221

[108] Xu WS, Parmigiani RB, Marks PA. Histone deacetylase inhibitors: Molecular mechanisms of action. Oncogene. 2007;**26**:5541-5552

[109] Richon VM, Sandhoff TW, Rifkind RA, Marks PA. Histone deacetylase inhibitor selectively induces p21 WAF1 expression and gene-associated histone acetylation. Proceedings of the National Academy of Sciences of the United States of America. 2000;**97**:1-6

[110] Sandor V, Senderowicz A, Mertins S, Sackett D, Sausville E, Blagoskonny MV, et al. P21-dependent G1 arrest with downregulation of cyclin D1 and upregulation of cyclin E by the histone deacetylase inhibitor FR901228. British Journal of Cancer. 2000;**83**:817-825

[111] Butler LM, Zhou X, Xu WS, Scher HI, Rifkind RA, Marks PA, et al. The histone deacetylase inhibitor SAHA arrests cancer cell growth, up-regulates thioredoxin-binding protein-2, and down-regulates thioredoxin. Proceedings of the National Academy of Sciences of the United States of America. 2002;**99**:11700-11705

[112] Frew AJ, Johnstone RW, Bolden JE. Enhancing the apoptotic and therapeutic effects of HDAC inhibitors. Cancer Letters. 2009;**280**:125-133

[113] Vrana J, Decker R, Johnson C, Wang Z, Jarvis W, Richon V, et al. Induction of apoptosis in U937 human leukemia cells by suberoylanilide hydroxamic acid (SAHA) proceeds through pathways that are regulated by Bcl-2/Bcl-XL, c-Jun, and p21CIP1, but independent of p53. Oncogene. 1999;**18**:7016-7025

[114] Nawrocki ST, Carew JS, Douglas L, Cleveland JL, Humphreys R, Houghton JA. Histone deacetylase inhibitors enhance lexatumumab-induced apoptosis via a p21 Cip1-dependent decrease in survivin levels. Cancer Research. 2007;**67**:6987-6995

[115] Harper JW, Adami GR, Wei N, Keyomarsi K, Elledge SJ. The p21 Cdk-interacting protein Cip1 is a potent inhibitor of G1 cyclin-dependent kinases. Cell. 1993;**75**:805-816

[116] Qiu L, Burgess A, Fairlie D, Leonard H, Parsons P, Gabrielli B. Histone deacetylase inhibitors trigger a G2 checkpoint in normal cells that is defective in tumor cells. Molecular Biology of the Cell. 2000;**11**:2069-2083

[117] Lee J, Choy ML, Ngo L, Foster SS, Marks PA. Histone deacetylase inhibitor induces DNA damage, which normal but not transformed cells can repair. Proceedings of the National Academy of Sciences of the United States of America. 2010;**107**:14639-14644

[118] Ruefli AA, Ausserlechner MJ, Bernhard D, Sutton VR, Tainton KM, Kofler R, et al. The histone deacetylase inhibitor and chemotherapeutic agent suberoylanilide hydroxamic acid (SAHA) induces a cell-death pathway characterized by cleavage of bid and production of reactive oxygen species. Proceedings of the National Academy of Sciences of the United States of America. 2001;**98**:10833-10838

[119] Rosato R, Almenara J, Dai Y, Grant S. Simultaneous activation of the intrinsic and extrinsic pathways by histone deacetylase (HDAC) inhibitors and tumor necrosis factor-related apoptosis-inducing ligand (TRAIL)

synergistically induces mitochondrial damage and apoptosis in human leukemia cells. Molecular Cancer Therapeutics. 2003;**2**:1273-1284

[120] Carlisi D, Lauricella M, D'Anneo A, Emanuele S, Angileri L, Di Fazio P, et al. The histone deacetylase inhibitor suberoylanilide hydroxamic acid sensitises human hepatocellular carcinoma cells to TRAIL-induced apoptosis by TRAIL-DISC activation. European Journal of Cancer. 2009;**45**:2425-2438

[121] Nakata S, Yoshida T, Horinaka M, Shiraishi T, Wakada M, Sakai T. Histone deacetylase inhibitors upregulate death receptor 5/TRAIL-R2 and sensitize apoptosis induced by TRAIL/APO2-L in human malignant tumor cells. Oncogene. 2004;**23**:6261-6271

[122] Fulda S, Küfer MU, Meyer E, van Valen F, Dockhorn-Dworniczak B, Debatin KM. Sensitization for death receptor- or drug-induced apoptosis by re-expression of caspase-8 through demethylation or gene transfer. Oncogene. 2001;**20**:5865-5877

[123] Ungerstedt JS, Sowa Y, Xu W, Shao Y, Dokmanovic M, Perez G, et al. Role of thioredoxin in the response of normal and transformed cells to histone deacetylase inhibitors. Proceedings of the National Academy of Sciences of the United States of America. 2005;**102**:673-678

[124] Li Z, Zhu WG. Targeting histone deacetylases for cancer therapy: From molecular mechanisms to clinical implications. International Journal of Biological Sciences. 2014;**10**:757-770

[125] Miller KM, Tjeertes JV, Coates J, Legube G, Polo SE, Britton S, et al. Human HDAC1 and HDAC2 function in the DNA-damage response to promote DNA nonhomologous end-joining. Nature Structural and Molecular Biology. 2010;**17**:1144-1151

[126] Bhaskara S, Knutson SK, Jiang G, Chandrasekharan MB, Wilson AJ, Zheng S, et al. Hdac3 is essential for the maintenance of chromatin structure and genome stability. Cancer Cell. 2010;**18**:436-447

[127] Thurn KT, Thomas S, Raha P, Qureshi I, Munster PN. Histone deacetylase regulation of ATM-mediated DNA damage signaling. Molecular Cancer Therapeutics. 2013;**12**:2078-2087

[128] Kao GD, McKenna WG, Guenther MG, Muschel RJ, Lazar MA, Yen TJ. Histone deacetylase 4 interacts with 53BP1 to mediate the DNA damage response. The Journal of Cell Biology. 2003;**160**:1017-1027

[129] Kotian S, Liyanarachchi S, Zelent A, Parvin JD. Histone deacetylase 9 and 10 are required for homologous recombination. The Journal of Biological Chemistry. 2011;**286**:7722-7726

[130] Gorospe M, de Cabo R. AsSIRTing the DNA damage response. Trends in Cell Biology. 2008;**18**:77-83

[131] Kaidi A, Weinert BT, Choudhary C, Jackson SP. Human SIRT6 promotes DNA end resection through CtIP deacetylation. Science. 2010;**329**:1348-1353

[132] Motoslavsky R, Chua KF, Lombard DB, Pang WW, Fischer MR, Gellon L, et al. Genomic instability and aging-like phenotype in the absence of mammalian SIRT6. Cell. 2006;**124**:315-329

[133] Rosato RR, Almenara JA, Grant S. The histone deacetylase inhibitor MS-275 promotes differentiation or apoptosis in human leukemia cells through a process regulated by generation of reactive oxygen species and induction of p21 CIP1/WAF1. Cancer Research. 2003;**63**:3637-3645

[134] Deroanne CF, Bonjean K, Servotte S, Devy L, Colige A, Clausse N, et al. Histone deacetylases inhibitors as anti-angiogenic agents altering vascular endothelial growth factor signaling. Oncogene. 2002;**21**:427-436

[135] Jeong JW, Bae MK, Ahn MY, Kim SH, Sohn TK, Bae MH, et al. Regulation and destabilization of HIF-1alpha by ARD1-mediated acetylation. Cell. 2002;**111**:709-720

[136] Pulukuri S, Gorantla B, Rao J. Inhibition of histone deacetylase activity promotes invasion of human cancer cells through activation of urokinase plasminogen activator. The Journal of Biological Chemistry. 2007;**282**:35594-35603

[137] Fournel M, Bonfils C, Hou Y, Yan P, Trachy-Bourget MC, Kalita A, et al. MGCD0103, a novel isotype-selective histone deacetylase inhibitor, has broad spectrum antitumor activity in vitro and in vivo. Molecular Cancer Therapeutics. 2008;**7**:759-768

[138] Vigushin DM, Ali S, Pace PE, Mirsaidi N, Ito K, Adcock I, et al. Trichostatin a is a histone deacetylase inhibitor with potent antitumor activity against breast cancer in vivo. Clinical Cancer Research. 2001;**7**:971-976

[139] Sato N, Ohta T, Kitagawa H, Kayahara M, Ninomiya I, Fushida S, et al. FR901228, a novel histone deacetylase inhibitor, induces cell cycle arrest and subsequent apoptosis in refractory human pancreatic cancer cells. International Journal of Oncology. 2004;**24**:679-685

[140] Kwon HJ, Owa T, Hassig CA, Shimada J, Schreiber SL. Depudecin induces morphological reversion of transformed fibroblasts via the inhibition of histone deacetylase. Proceedings of the National Academy of Sciences of the United States of America. 1998;**95**:3356-3361

[141] Mrakovcic M, Kleinheinz J, Fröhlich LF. Histone deacetylase inhibitor-induced autophagy in tumor cells: Implications for p53. International Journal of Molecular Sciences. 2017;**18**:1883

[142] Gammoh N, Lam D, Puente C, Ganley I, Marks PA, Jiang X. Role of autophagy in histone deacetylase inhibitor-induced apoptotic and nonapoptotic cell death. Proceedings of the National Academy of Sciences of the United States of America. 2012;**109**:6561-6565

[143] Carew JS, Nawrocki ST, Kahue CN, Zhang H, Yang C, Chung L, et al. Targeting autophagy augments the anticancer activity of the histone deacetylase inhibitor SAHA to overcome Bcr-Abl-mediated drug resistance. Blood. 2007;**110**:313-323

[144] Di Giacomo V, Di Valerio V, Rapino M, Bosco D, Cacciatore I, Ciulla M, et al. MRJF4, a novel histone deacetylase inhibitor, induces p21 mediated autophagy in PC3 prostate cancer cells. Cellular and Molecular Biology. 2015;**61**:17-23

[145] Wang J, Kim TH, Ahn MY, Lee J, Jung JH, Choi WS, et al. Sirtinol, a class III HDAC inhibitor, induces apoptotic and autophagic cell death in MCF-7 human breast cancer cells. International Journal of Oncology. 2012;**41**:1101-1109

[146] Shulak L, Beljanski V, Chiang C, Dutta SM, Van Grevenynghe J, Belgnaoui SM, et al. Histone deacetylase inhibitors potentiate vesicular stomatitis virus oncolysis in prostate cancer cells by modulating NF-kappa B-dependent autophagy. Journal of Virology. 2014;**88**:2927-2940

[147] Li J, Liu R, Lei Y, Wang K, Lau QC, Xie N, et al. Proteomic analysis revealed association of aberrant ROS signaling with suberoylanilide

hydroxamic acid-induced autophagy in Jurkat T-leukemia cells. Autophagy. 2010;**6**:711-724

[148] Long J, Zhao J, Yan Z, Liu Z, Wang N. Antitumor effects of a novel sulfur-containing hydroxamate histone deacetylase inhibitor H40. International Journal of Cancer. 2009;**124**:1235-1244

[149] Watanabe M, Adachi S, Matsubara H, Imai T, Yui Y, Mizushima Y. Induction of autophagy in malignant rhabdoid tumor cells by the histone deacetylase inhibitor FK228 through AIF translocation. International Journal of Cancer Research. 2009;**67**:55-67

[150] Zhang J, Ng S, Wang J, Zhou J, Tan S, Yang N, et al. Histone deacetylase inhibitors induce autophagy through FOXO1-dependent pathways. Autophagy. 2015;**11**:629-642

[151] Gandesiri M, Chakilam S, Ivanovska J, Benderska N, Ocker M, Di Fazio P, et al. DAPK plays an important role in panobinostat-induced autophagy and commits cells to apoptosis under autophagy deficient conditions. Apoptosis. 2012;**17**:1300-1315

[152] Ellis L, Bots M, Lindemann RK, Bolden JE, Newbold A, Cluse LA, et al. The histone deacetylase inhibitors LAQ824 and LBH589 do not require death receptor signaling or a functional apoptosome to mediate tumor cell death or therapeutic efficacy. Blood. 2009;**114**:380-393

[153] Sun W, Yi Y, Xia G, Zhao Y, Yu Y, Li L, et al. Nrf2-miR-129-3p-mTOR axis controls an miRNA regulatory network involved in HDACi-induced autophagy. Molecular Therapy. 2019;**27**:1039-1050

[154] Stankov MV, El Khatib M, Kumar Thakur B, Heitmann K, Panayotova-Dimitrova D, Schoening J, et al. Histone deacetylase inhibitors induce apoptosis in myeloid leukemia by suppressing autophagy. Leukemia. 2014;**28**:577-588

[155] Maccallum SF, Groves MJ, James J, Murray K, Appleyard V, Prescott AR, et al. Dysregulation of autophagy in chronic lymphocytic leukemia with the small-molecule sirtuin inhibitor tenovin-6. Scientific Reports. 2013;**3**:1275

[156] Fröhlich LF, Mrakovcic M, Smole C, Lahiri P, Zatloukal K. Epigenetic silencing of apoptosis-inducing gene expression can be efficiently overcome by combined SAHA and TRAIL treatment in uterine sarcoma cells. PLoS One. 2014;**9**:e91558

[157] Shao Y, Gao Z, Marks PA, Jiang X. Apoptotic and autophagic cell death induced by histone deacetylase inhibitors. Proceedings of the National Academy of Sciences of the United States of America. 2004;**101**:18030-18035

[158] Liu YL, Yang PM, Shun CT, Wu MS, Weng JR, Chen CC. Autophagy potentiates the anti-cancer effects of the histone deacetylase inhibitors in hepatocellular carcinoma. Autophagy. 2010;**6**:1057-1065

[159] Chiao M, Cheng W, Yang Y, Shen C, Chiao M, Cheng W, et al. Suberoylanilide hydroxamic acid (SAHA) causes tumor growth slowdown and triggers autophagy in glioblastoma stem cells. Autophagy. 2013;**9**:1509-1526

[160] El-Khoury V, Pierson S, Szwarcbart E, Brons NHC, Roland O, Cherrier-De Wilde S, et al. Disruption of autophagy by the histone deacetylase inhibitor MGCD0103 and its therapeutic implication in B-cell chronic lymphocytic leukemia. Leukemia. 2014;**28**:1636-1646

[161] Ahn MY, Ahn JW, Kim HS, Lee J, Yoon JH. Apicidin inhibits cell growth by downregulating IGF-1R in salivary mucoepidermoid carcinoma cells. Oncology Reports. 2015;**33**:1899-1907

[162] Hui KF, Yeung PL, Chiang AKS. Induction of MAPK- and ROS-dependent autophagy and apoptosis in gastric carcinoma by combination of romidepsin and bortezomib. Oncotarget. 2015;**7**:1-14

[163] Zhan Y, Gong K, Chen C, Wang H, Li W. P38 MAP kinase functions as a switch in MS-275-induced reactive oxygen species-dependent autophagy and apoptosis in human colon cancer cells. Free Radical Biology and Medicine. 2012;**53**:532-543

[164] Park EY, Woo Y, Kim SJ, Kim DH, Lee EK, De U, et al. Anticancer effects of a new SIRT inhibitor, MHY2256, against human breast cancer MCF-7 cells via regulation of MDM2-p53 binding. International Journal of Biological Sciences. 2016;**12**:1555-1567

[165] Fröhlich LF, Mrakovcic M, Smole C, Zatloukal K. Molecular mechanism leading to SAHA-induced autophagy in tumor cells: Evidence for a p53-dependent pathway. Cancer Cell International. 2016;**16**:1-15

[166] Sykes SM, Mellert HS, Holbert MA, Li K, Lane WS, Mcmahon SB. Acetylation of the p53 DNA binding domain regulates apoptosis induction. Molecular Cell. 2006;**24**:841-851

[167] Tang Y, Luo J, Zhang W. Tip60-dependent acetylation of p53 modulates the decision between cell-cycle arrest and apoptosis. Molecular Cell. 2006;**24**:827-839

[168] Barlev NA, Liu L, Chehab NH, Mansfield K, Harris KG, Halazonetis TD, et al. Acetylation of p53 activates transcription through recruitment of coactivators/histone acetyltransferases. Molecular Cell. 2001;**8**:1243-1254

[169] Luo J, Li M, Tang Y, Laszkowska M, Roeder RG, Gu W. Acetylation of p53 augments its site-specific DNA binding both in vitro and in vivo. Proceedings of the National Academy of Sciences of the United States of America. 2003;**101**:2259-2264

[170] Zhao Y, Lu S, Wu L, Chai G, Wang H, Chen Y, et al. Acetylation of p53 at lysine 373/382 by the histone deacetylase inhibitor depsipeptide induces expression of p21 Waf1/Cip1. Molecular and Cellular Biology. 2006;**26**:2782-2790

[171] Seo SK, Jin HO, Woo SH, Kim YS, An S, Lee JH, et al. Histone deacetylase inhibitors sensitize human non-small cell lung cancer cells to ionizing radiation through acetyl p53-mediated c-myc down-regulation. Journal of Thoracic Oncology. 2011;**6**:1313-1319

[172] Mrakovcic M, Bohner L, Hanisch M, Fröhlich LF. Epigenetic targeting of autophagy via HDAC inhibition in tumor cells: Role of p53. International Journal of Molecular Sciences. 2018;**19**:3952

[173] Hrzenjak A, Moinfar F, Kremser ML, Strohmeier B, Petru E, Zatloukal K, et al. Histone deacetylase inhibitor vorinostat suppresses the growth of uterine sarcomas in vitro and in vivo. Molecular Cancer. 2010;**9**:49

[174] De U, Son JY, Sachan R, Park YJ, Kang D, Yoon K, et al. A new synthetic histone deacetylase inhibitor, MHY2256, induces apoptosis and autophagy cell death in endometrial cancer cells via p53 acetylation. International Journal of Molecular Sciences. 2018;**19**:2743